Secrets to

Ageless Health

and Beauty

(How to Stay 10 Steps Ahead of the Aging Process)

Renatta McCoy Baker

Health is real wealth, without it we are unable to pay life's debt, which is the price to be paid to live an abundant life. ~Renatta

Renatta Translation: Reborn, Rebirth To Create New Again

Meet the Author/Coach/Trainer

Hello I am Coach Renatta, I am 48 years young and loving my life that God granted me access to. I am a wife and mother of three who has lived a holistic healthy lifestyle that has sustained my health and wellbeing through life's many ups and downs. After working years in the Information Technology industry I decided to follow my natural inclination and passion for sharing and promoting health and wellness with the world to transform lives. In 2015, I became certified in personal training and set off on my health and healing crusade, with a plan to personally help as many people as I could in support of their health and wellness journeys. I realized trading time to personally reach people had its challenges and limitations with impacting the masses.

In 2017 Ree Ree Fitness has grown from a small training fitness boutique to an ultimate health and wellness company that offers nutritional support, lifestyle coaching, books and videos.

My 5 year goal plan for my business is to help 10,000 women and men successfully live out their highest quality of life via my signature health and fitness brand. I believe our true destiny is cumulative of every path we have journeyed. There is really no real destination in life besides death. When one journey ends another begins it continues until our lifecycle is completed and we transition back to our ultimate source of being. Many people may experience the challenges and struggles of weight loss, finding or becoming the perfect mate, deciding on a rewarding career, walking the journey of forgiveness down to discovering our true life's passion. The larger journey is the long winding road with all the detours, wrong directions, stop signs, red lights, speed bumps, dead ends, changing lanes, getting off the beaten path to finding ourselves. The health and wellness journey as all other journeys many times shed light on deeper issues that we uncover during our pilgrimage to self-discovery and self-awareness.

Our journeys allow us to look at life from a broader view and serves to awaken our soul and mind and give our struggles and successes meaning. The work we do in this lifetime on ourselves is the most important and the hardest work we will ever do on this planet. We are able to tap into our self-reliance, self-realization, self-actualization, self-belief, self-love, self-respect, self-worth, self-confidence and make no mistake by no means loving "thyself" considered selfish. The encompassing journey of self is simply called LIFE!

Preface

At 48 I often run into old friends, classmates and former colleagues after years and the recurring theme was how I seem to be aging backwards. The "Wow you have not aged a bit, what are you doing to stay so young?" In the few moments of brief conversation, I try to extend my appreciation for their kind words and share my healthy lifestyle mantras. There is never enough time to sufficiently convey the helpful tips that could also be of benefit to their lifestyle. As the conversations added up about the many ways I strive to live a healthy lifestyle blueprint by exercising, healthy eating and employing preventive methods to gain a few steps in front of good old father time, the thought would arise to write a book. I finally decided to write it down, make it plain for any and every one who wanted to learn in more depth about optimal health strategies to live in the highest echelons of life which is "Total Health and Wellness".

I always knew I would write a book on health and wellness. I was very sure of the "WHY" but unsure on the "HOW" to present all the information and make it as comprehensive as possible. I really wanted people to absorb it, process it and make it applicable to their daily lives. I wanted to ensure the information did not get lost in translation or fall on death ears with deep terminology and medical statistics. In addition, I wanted to share real health information and step out of the box of all the health and fitness jargon that exist in the social media realm of buzz words, hashtags, the 30/60/90 day challenge mentality. I did not want to write an entire book on exercises from A to Z or how to get a six-pack by summer (2nd book in the making), but I knew I wanted to share and present health and wellness on a deeper latitudinous scale and not just focus on fitness in of itself.

I had envisioned writing a book outlining how to incorporate healthy habits, information that extends far beyond the gym workout, latest diet plan, workout attire or discussions about whether cardio is superior or inferior versus resistance training for fat loss. Fitness has taken on all sorts of viewpoints, arguments and debates about what diet or exercise routine is the best which changes per each expert, armature opinion and arm chair fitness enthusiast. So many times I've witnessed conversation after conversation, fitness rhetoric and daily social media postings on fitness without any real mentions holistic health to maintain the vitality of life itself. The objective of true health is all about sustaining life in the healthiest vein. I have seen gimmick after gimmick promised, promoted and sold to the highest quick fix junkie bidder from the suck it in waist-trainer movement to the typical hot product push demanding you to "drink green drinks and meal replacements to create your dream body by summer", to the risky fitness stunts or crazy workouts videos of a popular celebrity trainer or social media proclaimed health and fitness model only done for the sake of social media purposes. There wasn't and still not much substantial information on how to live a well-balanced healthy lifestyle. There is no shortage of fitness post with well-planned pictures and hashtags that spawn the "The Get Fit for Summer Now" frenzy. Health and wellness is typically pushed aside while the "Grind and Bear It" mentality "Beast or Die" takes over souls like zombies. The fact is, it's perfectly fine to tap into your beast mode on a needed basis however, we all should know when to cycle on and off and when to rest, recover and relax. So I wanted to contribute my part or my truth as it relates to real health.

I felt compelled to provide information on lifestyle changes that would add quality years to your life versus focusing on being fit at any cost or going all in for a temporary fix. Focusing solely on one desired body part (Abs, Glutes and Guns) is not a comprehensive viewpoint of healthy living. We live life 365 days a year that is if you are fortunate enough not to be voted off the island for lack of a better way to phrase nobody makes it out alive.

It was crystal clear that I wanted to present true health and wellness as the foundation of living well and how to continually tap into your very own reservoir of "Fountain of Youth". The very core of living well is about preserving the body inside out to include Mind, Body and Soul.

They say there is no such thing as a SECRET, This may be true but what is hidden in plain sight becomes a secret to you...
~ Renatta

Acknowledgments

I give all praises to my Lord and Savior for my life and allowing me to live a happy, healthy abundant blessed life. I wake up every day and give thanks to God Almighty! It means nothing without God who has blessed me to be sound in my Mind, Body and Spirit. HALLELUJAH!!! Thank You Lord!..........

To My Mother: My health blueprint was handed down by my mother, which was handed down by her father. A mother's love extends deep like the roots of the tree of life. To my beautiful ageless spirit mother who taught me in so many ways the true meaning of strength, health and grace under fire. My mother imparted healthy eating and holistic health as I grew to understand how very important it was and always will be to take the best care of myself. The many days I thought I suffered not being able to eat the sugar cereals and the fast foods my friends enjoyed while growing up. Reminiscing back to the trips to the health food store walking down the aisles smelling the natural earthly produce of which I thought yuck!!!! Aisle after aisle no cookies and ice cream in sight. I can recall wishing for the hamburger patty special sauce lettuce, onions, cheese, tomatoes and the golden fries that glistened with salt from the yellow arches that left grease stains on the red carton with a good old brown colored fizzy soda pop to wash it all down. How I remember that good ole soda fizz burn and the gulp that always followed. But my mother's agenda served to be a true blessing as those days are still imprinted like a long lasting fingerprint on my brain that reads "Healthy Is Best". Thank you Lady Jewell for leaving me the gem of all gems my healthy blue print that lives inside me forever. I Love you Mom ALWAYS!!!

To My Father: My first superhero I knew I called father, the man who taught me to be an independent thinker and use my own logic and intellect constructively when approaching life's many challenges. I would say I am a daddy's girl. My dad gifted me with my propensity to be physically and mentally strong. The very first person I ever saw lifting a bar of weights. Thank you for never saying NO to my many request for chocolate covered almond ice crème from Highs. My mental toughness was developed through your insights of how to mentally survive in a tough world. I now look back on those many conversation and talks and realized that it helped me to create my mental blueprint. I always looked to my father to provide me with sound advice and guidance through many of my tough situations on my life's journey. Your advice and knowledge will always and forever be priceless. Thanks Dad!!! I love and appreciate you more than you will ever know.

To My Husband: My marathon love, my behind the scenes number one supporter, the real MVP who keeps my diet in check, my personal chef, my accountability life partner, puts up with my sporadic moments of insanity of 2:00am handstand pushups, my real life Super Man. I can't accept all the credit for my strength as my husband has been my rock of Gibraltar for 22 years and counting. He saves me from myself, his patience, kindness and understanding beyond comprehension has inspired me on countless days when I wanted to throw in the towel. Thanks Husband! I Love Love Love you!!!! My Eternal Mate, My God Send and my Bless Up!

To My Children: My A'yanna Jewell and My Christian Vaughn and My angel baby Laila Angelic. As parents we are our children's true heroes. No cape needed only unconditional love and support for our children. Our children look to us for guidance and strength we are their first role models rightfully so. Parents are important as we set the tone for their excellence, how to love, how to forgive and how to approach life matters. My children are my whole entire heart beat and world, my reasons and motivation to keep going and going. I want to live this life for as long as God will keep me to watch my children live out their dreams and reach their goals and be healthy productive citizens and live abundant lives with their children. It is not the material things we give our children that proves to be invaluable in life even after death. It is the example we set and our time as they watch and learn which provides them the foundation to replicate and extend for generations beyond.

To My Friends and Family: They say those who are willing to support and follow you for who you are without having to persuade, cajole, beguile and beg. Those that gravitate towards your inner authentic self are your tribe, your village and well-spring. There is no need to convince people when genuine friendships have been mutually and respectfully established. A big thank you, to all who have supported my health crusade at its grassroots conception when it was just me sharing my daily health and gym post and you all recognized my natural proclivity of inspiring others through living a healthy lifestyle.

Thank you for fanning the flame and allowing me to inspire you! As you have watered my seeds of passion and filled my bucket.

To All of You: To all who purchased this book who have now become a part of my extended family tribe. Thank you!!! Moreover, thank you for moving forward in living a healthier lifestyle and taking care of the person who matters the most YOU! Thank You for your generosity and buying this book. I hope you will find the content useful and as you learn I hope you will share it

forward with others to inspire change in their lives as well.
THINK WELL.... EAT WELL.... LIVE WELL
.... BE BLESSED!

Last But Not Least! To Me: It is very important to recognize your own resolve and push through to the person you are becoming. The many nights I doubted whether people would want to read a book about true health and wellness and thought people are only really interested in changing their body on a physical level. I have to thank myself for not faltering and pushing forward seeing the vision clear and just started writing and following through to fruition.

In Memoriam

This book is dedicated to my brother David R. McCoy
~ To Rest is Heaven (09.17.1967 – 03.01.2018) ~

Contents

Introduction

Congratulations!!!!!!! You have taken the first step and invested wisely in your health by purchasing this book. Changing small daily habits yield big rewards and pays off in more energy, mental clarity, managing weight loss, flawless skin, strong hair and nails, a strong healthy mind, soul and the list goes on and on. I will stop for all practical reasons due to the fact I am so excited to share more benefits in the following chapters to come. Let's get started!

This book is not your average "How to Diet", "Count Calories or "Stressing Over the Number on the Scale" reflected in pounds smiling smugly up at you. Besides the scale has bullied you and given you a misplaced preoccupation with scale weight far too long. The information in this book will far outweigh pounds on a scale. You will not find the latest and greatest trendy yo-yo diet or unrealistic strength training for mortal combat workout here. This book will not be focused primarily on weight loss at any cost at the expense of being healthy in of itself. It is not the "How to be Skinny" book nor am I trying to sell, promote or sponsor any product, pill or drink that promises instant weight loss and abs that magically appear out of thin air. As a matter of fact, this book won't promise you anything at all about weight loss.

This book is for anybody who wants to take their health and wellness in their own hands and become their own best advocate for adopting a healthier lifestyle. It is for those who want to create sustained health and improve their quality of life on a daily basis. If you want to transform your health blueprint this book is for you.

My intention with this book is to transform your current mindset in and around health while expanding your knowledge of wellness. True health is not about temporary diets, extreme exercising, a particular body shape or the block formation shape of abdominals. It serves to refocus on optimal health and not just the aesthetics of the body, dress or jean size or the number on a scale. The objective here is to inform and teach you overall about the body as a full functioning, well-oiled machine (the greatest machine ever invented). Allow this book to guide you, to inspire you to learn more about how your body functions in addition to the food and strategies necessary to maintain optimal health as you age. Keep it in your car, keep a copy at the office, keep it at your fingertips when you are making a trip to the grocery store. Let it serve as your go to book. I pray this book will not only find you but meet you where you are, irrespective to what your personal health and wellness goals and journey may be. I also hope it can reach you in other areas of your life. Do not confuse health and wellness as the ultimate journey. There is no doubt our mind, our soul and our bodies are the prerequisites of living a fully purposed life of not simply existing. LIFE is our ultimate journey where you leave your footprints in the sand. Health and wellness allows you to make those foot prints for years to come. The sand will always find its way under the feet of a healthy soul.

As I think back on my own thoughts of what it means to be healthy, my thoughts and beliefs have changed tremendously over the years. At the tender age of 18 being young and gifted with wonderful genetics and a torch metabolism I believed I was as healthy as my jeans looked on my size zero frame. I did not have to work hard to maintain my weight it was never anything I gave a second thought. Well as life often has the last word, we are not young forever. As my life progressed and I lived long enough to see loved ones and friends stricken with debilitating degenerative diseases and illness my mindset changed from the once invincible 18 year old who felt immune to sickness and disease, who looked at health as simply being privileged to shop off of the size 0-2 racks. I thought hey I am small means I'm healthy right? My 40 something year old self knows enough now and understands health does not necessarily correspond to a specific size or look. I also now realize we may not be able to predict our future down the road but, we can wake up daily with deliberate intention and resolve to make healthier lifestyle adjustments that bring forth wellness in all areas of life.

My efforts to remain healthy and youthful are at the forefront of my daily life practices. So if you ask me today right now, at the tender wise age of 48 what my definition of being healthy means? I would undoubtedly tell you it is not just being physically fit to perform a certain activity or looking great in a two piece bikini for a hashtag season. I would tell you being healthy encompasses the mind, soul, body from the inside out. Real health considers your thoughts. Real health considers your self-esteem. Real health considers our ability to cultivate loving relationships including our most important relationships with God and self.

So first off, about those SECRETS.....there are absolutely no hidden secrets to being healthy and fit, it is already within you. It is going to take relearning what you think you know about health, wellness and aging. You have everything you need to change your lifestyle by redirecting your thought process and forming habitual healthy habits that will produce real substantial change in your life. The mind is powerful it is our foundation for everything we attract in our lives. The mind attracts either good or bad depending on what you focus your attention on and feed your thoughts. There is our conscious mind but we also have our subconscious mind. The two are very important in seeing real results and transformation in our lives. The conscious mind can be clear on our goals and objectives. The subconscious is always hungry and has so much potential to sabotage many of our hard earned efforts. Always be mindful to guard your thoughts, what you read, view, listen, give attention to and the words you speak. The subconscious mind has no quality checks and balances it does not qualify, discern, or pick and choose it accepts everything. BE MINDFUL!!!!

So you decided it's time to jump start your health. Maybe you have put it off over and over to a point you are finally serious enough to act NOW. Good for you! We all tend to procrastinate when we feel we are not ready to acknowledge and address deeper issues that require some serious thought, process, duration of time and actions on our part to do real work. By virtue of deciding to purchase this book you have opened yourself up to learning more about how to preserve and maintain your overall health and wellness.

I believe this book will equip you with the tools to tap into your power within and support you in making more informed healthy choices. I also wholeheartedly believe when you provide people with the information you empower them with opportunities to change and build upon new ideas to grow, learn and ultimately evolve. It is my intent with this book to spark the fire that God has already lit when he created you even before your ultimate journey of life began on this earth. I am just a catalyst here to fan the flames no matter how deep down or buried it may be today. Allow due process for learning new concepts, take it one day at a time and live in the process of accepting and implementing change. Don't try to manipulate your results by trying to rush and hurry up your AFTER. Everybody loves the after results photo, but everybody hates the process or what is known as our 'In the meantime".

That place our in the "In the Meantime" is our cocoon of transformation it is where the magic happens. Your "In the Process" is shaping your "Inner Wherewithal", it is teaching you "Inner Strength" comes from deep within. Sure we build our bodies strong but our spirit should be stronger. Our mind should become a strong force field the breaks the chains of complacent thinking.

Change will make you feel uncomfortable at first until it because second nature or a habit. That nagging uncomfortable feeling is your mind fighting complacency. First you have to CARE enough to COMMIT to doing the WORK. CHANGE your daily habits and FIGHT COMPLACENCY EVERYDAY. Let's Go!!!

Chapter 1

The Proverbial Forever 25 Syndrome

Blow Out Your Candles .....Blow Up Your Balloons .....Eat the Cake..... Celebrate the Blessing of Every Second, Every Minute, Every Day and Every Year of Life....

There was a time in our lives when the hip-hip hoorays and whohoooo's of our birthday meant a time for fun and celebration. As children, right next to Christmas we looked forward with anticipation of celebrating another birthday. I mean who doesn't love a party, the gifts, being the center of attention to celebrate our beautiful existence in life? We would anxiously tell everybody we knew and anybody inclined to listen that we were looking forward to celebrating another year of life. There was a time in life we could tell our age with pride and joy without feeling down about growing older.

By the time we hit our 25th anniversary of life our enthusiasm to share our birthday starts to diminish. We no longer share those birthday alerts with the same enthusiasm. The hip-hip-hoorays and whohooo's morphed into anxieties and Ohhhhh Noooooo's!!!!! After 25 the whole conversation about age becomes classified personal information reserved only for flashing our driver's license on a needed basis.

As our borndays start to add up in years and we can no longer count our age on our fingers and toes, our birthdays start to remind us that we are aging and it pulls our mortality coat tail. We all know that getting older is a blessing however, it is natural to ponder death as it is a part of every human's lifecycle. No one lives forever. But let's focus our attention on the life we have now. Although no one can ever predict the day or hour, you can live fully in the NOW! Now is all we really have, live abundantly now. The truth is, from our very first breath of life the aging process sets in. But aging should be regarded as a necessary passage that symbolizes one of our biggest blessings (LIVING). Unfortunately, we tend to associate negative images and stereotypes about the aging process. Society socializes us to believe getting older has its harsh realities of weight gain, memory loss, poor eyesight, gray hairs, walking canes, wheelchairs, oxygen tanks, ostomy bags, nursing homes and finally death. Yes that is a pretty bleak and frightening outlook I'd say. Stop! Who says we have to surrender to these negative ideas about living a long fruitful life. I must say if I held these beliefs about aging I would be hesitant, reluctant and fearful of aging as well. It is a good thing I do not hold this mindset about longevity, aging and borndays. I practice loving my life through all chapters and seasons.

Of course another year of life means we did not die which is the blessing that another year adds. Where we once informed people of our birthday, when we passed that golden ripe age that everybody holds in their mind (an imaginary line of demarcation) between being considered old versus young birthdays become silent vigils. For some we stop alerting others of our birthdays if we do, we may skim a year or two off our real age and hope nobody realizes or has the time to do the math or has a calculator on hand.

Youth and beauty are used interchangeably. When we look back on our youth it was a time most likely we looked and felt our best. Maybe a time we fell in love or a time we felt free without fear or a time where our energy levels matched our big dreams. Living a life of longevity should be viewed with appreciation and gratitude. Everyone is not given the blessing of living a long healthy life be grateful for each year you get to celebrate living.

I have great news!!!! This book will share with you preventive measures, tactical information on how to manage even delay the wrinkles, saggy skin, dentures, age spots, aches, pains, weight gain, memory loss and much more. First things first, wipe out all the bad images and beliefs about growing older and reprogram your mind with positive images of aging and living your best quality of life every day. Growing older does not have to be feared or viewed as the other scarlet letter "A" for AGING. Become not only inspired by life but by living a life filled with love and happiness that you designed with the powers of your thoughts. When you shift your thoughts and views on living an abundant long quality life, you give yourself every opportunity to age gracefully with peace of mind. Longevity is not granted to everyone who makes an appearance on earth. As a matter of fact, just because you show up on earth does not mean you show up in your life. Showing up in life requires action and in that action, life transforms into real living. Real beauty is not what you look like on the outside contrary to popular belief. The beauty of life is the awareness and knowing that God gave you everything you need to solve every problem in this world. For every issue in life there is a prayer, grace, mercy, a well-defined action plan and execution for resolution that leads to an ultimate solution.

You must work daily on creating a healthy mindset about everything you do in life. You don't just work on your lifestyle for a summer season. You must work on your mind through all seasons of life. This is also true about your thoughts on getting older, losing or maintaining your weight, your current circumstances, to believing in your own ability to create the best versions of "YOU". I say versions because it's a continuous process of self-improvement. Do not listen to what the world says about aging or this metaphoric over the hill hog wash. There does not have to be an imaginary hill. Your life's terrain can be smooth flat land no age hills to speak of. Society does not define you. Reprogram your thoughts to reshape your paradigm and your life will align with every good thought you feed it. Once you are in full control of your mindset your perception can be adjusted, to view the aging process as being something you manage, control and appreciate.

Have you ever wondered why someone looks 10 years younger than their natural born chronological age? Do you stop to think when you run into an old friend that you seem to be aging faster than your peers? Have you met a person twice your age but look years younger? Our first thoughts are some people just lucked up with great genetics. Sure we are all dealt a hand with our genetics which some are born with winning hands while others may have to shuffle more cards from the deck. We all want the glitter dust of youth some are just born with a little more than others this does not preclude anyone from looking their best and living a healthier lifestyle at any age. Asking questions about how to age gracefully is great but if not met with a daily action plan, aging gracefully will always remain a rhetorical question and whimsical wishing and hoping to look younger.

I am excited to share with you information and health tips to activate and tap into your very own fountain of youth. Since you are still reading up until this point, I guess I have peaked your interest and curiosity in hearing more on how to navigate the maze of health and wellness as it relates to aging. This book is designed to assist you on how to connect your mind, your soul and your body to boost your overall quality of life. Ok "25" may have been a great age for you but I am here to say being healthy and fit exist at any age don't leave your best self behind. Your best self is always a work in progress. To be brutally honest there is no such reality of your best self. All that exist is deep daily introspection and reflection that should lead us to continuous improvement in all areas of our lives. Ask yourself this! If 2017 is your best year, does this mean all subsequent years thereafter will be your worst years of existence? Does this mean you will never have a great year beyond the year you proclaimed as your BEST year of life? If you reached your goal weight does this mean you can now stop living healthy and let yourself slip back into your old habits? If you got married does this mean your wedding day is the best day that will ever exist as a married couple? You set yourself up for not embracing the thought that each day should get better and better. Don't put your BEST anything (day, life, body, self) in a box to be lived on a one time only basis.

You are selling yourself short when you try to convince yourself there is a best life at a certain age, weight, chapter in your life or marital status. Your Best Life is happening Now!!!! The prevailing thought and focus should be in terms of how to live an inspired life everyday this adds up to the greatest life lived in spite of many life's ups and downs.

Chapter 2

Gravity, Genetics and Aging

Gravity says: "I last forever"....Genetics says: "Doesn't matter I can't be changed".... Age says: "Hush God left me in charge"............

When we speak about aging unfortunately, there are many variables out of our control. The 3 variables are: age, gravity and genetics. The first two (age and gravity) pretty much are a constant in the continuous lifecycle. We are unable to control the force that the nature of gravity exacts on our bodies. Well actually there is one way to control the force of both gravity and age and that is to die. Death stops age and gravity immediately. Genetics play a vital role in how we tend to age however, we are able to manipulate certain aspects of our genetics which we are not as fortunate to do with age and gravity. We may not be able to see it...feel it...eat it...or touch gravity but it is always there. The constant down pulling of gravity takes its toll on every part of our body. We need to really understand this force of nature and what it does to our bodies every second, minute, hour, day and years we live.

Let's take a look at our spine. Our spine consists of vertebrae and sponge like disc. Gravity pulls downward causing the discs to lose moisture throughout the day, and we actually get a bit shorter at the end of the day. So when we go to sleep at night, the sleep process returns the moisture overnight but not 100%. This is why as we age we seem to shrink and get shorter over our lifetime. It is clear to see why we should not cheat the number of hours of quality sleep. The sleep process rejuvenates all of our body's functions. In addition, water is very important to aid in the sleep recovery process. Drink a glass of room temperature water before bed each night to help restore your body during the resting phase.

The height we lose due to gravity's pull wreaks havoc on the rest of our bodies as well. Our organs become compressed. Gravity pushing downward expands our waist without even physically eating. The nick name for that extra weight around our waist, is affectionately known as our "Love Handles". However, the proper medical term for love handles, are "Compression Wrinkles" because they are in part a direct result of compression of the spine due to "Gravity". Who would think to link gravity to an expanding waistline? Not many people including myself. So don't be too hard on yourself if those few inches are not budging even after exercising and clean eating habits. It's pretty difficult to beat gravity at its own game.

The old saying goes "What goes up must come down" is a very true statement. As we age gravity takes its toll on the circulatory system as well. It is very important for blood to pump freely through our veins and arteries. Gravity will slow this process resulting in blocked arteries, varicose veins, and swollen limbs. The heart has to work harder over time. Over our lifespan our most critical organs tend to eventually wear out. Eating foods that prevent clogged arteries helps the heart to pump blood freely and lessens the effects of gravity's impact on circulation.

It's easy to see how gravity impacts our body externally. Everybody has witnessed their body changing, a sag or wrinkle here and there and maybe some extra jiggle in places we never had before. People are quick to seek out easy fixes and forgo the life long process of healthy living. This is why plastic surgery has become so popular these days. There are tons of people who are not interested in living a holistic lifestyle they want the instant gratification that surgery brings. Let's get back to the effects gravity wreaks on our bodies. As we age our organs begin to prolapse, or shift from their rightful place in our body. The organs in our bodies become less efficient. Common issues are bladder, kidney and digestive problems due to prolapsed organs. In fact for centuries, yoga practitioners have performed hand stands to help realign the organs in the body due to gravity. I myself employ yoga to help with the effects of gravity on my short stature.

I am petite enough so I fight gravity every chance I get. As the old saying goes "If you can't beat 'em join 'em", well I would not typically join an adversary however, gravity is an unformidable opponent so it's better to simultaneously work with and against gravity at the same time. Don't get down about gravity (pun intended). We may not be able to control gravity however, when we perform certain exercise it becomes an invisible force that our bodies can use as resistance training. You can fight gravity by performing exercises that requires you to jump up and down such as "Rebounding" which is an exercise technique where you are jumping on a trampoline for a specified period of time. It is one of my favorite fun exercises I perform. Rebounding promotes cleansing of the lymphatic system as well. A few more of my personal favorite exercises are jumping rope and jump squats all of these exercises are great ways to cross train against gravity's pull. Swimming is an excellent exercise as well. Also try adding Yoga to your current workout regimen. My favorite way to cross train against gravity pull are handstand pushups, yoga and jumping on my trampoline. There are many yoga poses that take gravity into consideration and conditions the body to age slower through focused breathing, meditation, concentration and strengthening poses.

Chapter 3

Know Thy Self (The ABC's of U)

The Most Important Letter in the Alphabet is 'U"........

You may be asking yourself where do I start on the journey to completely loving myself? Have you taken the time to learn who you really are at the very core of your soul? Not the representative that shows up to handle business or the contrived public image but, the real you behind the veil. The person without the makeup, the nicely coiffed manicured hair, the designer wardrobe, painted finger nails, titles, the false pride, our fears, shame, self-doubt and insecurities. We all have the person who is tucked away under those many layers of false identities. Many people build a wall even for themselves to prevent being vulnerable to real self-awareness and self-growth. So we try to replace that person with a painted face, a number on a scale, a dress size, marital status, social status, and get caught between the façade of image versus our inner person. This dynamic is even more prevalent in the social media spectrum. Many people are losing their identities to image driven social networks that perpetuate alter egos and images of a perfect life. Let us continue to explore ways to undercover our real true authentic self. The fact is we are a composite of everything in our lives good, bad and indifferent. Whether we like it or not it is our lot in life or our cause to bear. We are not just all the good things that happened to us and we should never define ourselves by a particular circumstance or incident that adversely affected our lives. You will be better served defining yourself by the strength and courage it took for you to overcome and triumph whatever situation and struggle life dealt you. Unfortunately, when we are hurt we turn to our alter ego and pride as a coping mechanism to try and prevent future hurt and pain from penetrating our heart again. Most people live guarded and suspicious of everybody and everything as a result of past hurt. Put aside all the superficial surface trappings like who you think people really want to see, this prevents us from really getting to know ourselves intimately down to our spirit. Take time to understand your personal self-health blue print you created over the years. Ask yourself questions surrounding how you process your joy, pains, fears, doubts and give yourself real intimate feedback. Of course we all know things like our favorite color and what we love to eat and enjoy but can you answer real pertinent questions about yourself and your health? Below are some essential questions to ponder.

- Do you know your blood type?
- Are you predispose or have a family history of cancer(s)?
- Do you know your cholesterol levels?
- When was the last time you had an annual check-up?
- Do you ignore your health issues?
- How do you tend to deal with stress?
- What technique do you employ to help manage everyday stressors?
- Are you ashamed of some things that happened in your past?
- Are you afraid people will define you by your mistakes?
- How do you deal with hurt and pain and betrayal?
- Have you had your thyroid checked?

- Is it easy for you to celebrate others but hard to celebrate yourself?
- What is your body type? How do you tend to lose or gain weight?
- Are you an emotional eater?
- Do you become anxious about the future?
- Are you a fixer? Do you take on other's burdens?
- Do you feel unworthy?
- Do you constantly put other's needs before your own?
- Do you beat yourself up for making a mistake(s)?
- Have you forgiven yourself for those mistakes in life?
- Are you holding on to things from childhood that you feel ashamed of?
- Has there been any form of abuse in your childhood, or as an adult that you try to mask the pain with food?

These are just a few questions you should ask yourself the answers will help you become more aware of how you deal with your overall health. We underestimate the role stress and unresolved issues play in our lives. Stress beats our chronological age to the punch. Before your birthday even shows up on the calendar stress will have aged you more than your natural born birthdate.

Knowing vital and key information about your health and being proactive in a preventive mode puts you ahead of the curb of any unforeseen issues that may present themselves later on in life. When we are proactive with our health it gives us an advantage of staying ahead of life's uncertainties. Some of life's twist and turns can be managed and even reversed if caught early enough as a result of practicing preventative measures. Be mindful keep those annual health appointments, do the monthly breast exams do not ignore those persistent aches and pains. It is better to err on the side of caution and prevention than to allow issues to slip through the cracks. Stay the course and on top of your health first, everything else gets runner up 2nd place.

Many of us tend to be emotional eaters. We give food power and control over our lives. Food is a staple of most social gatherings, wedding celebrations, date nights, girl's night out and all the late night couch potato movie binges. We feel we need food at the center of attention and our world. Food makes us feel good when we are going through life's ups and downs. I am an emotional eater I have been known to get the warm and fuzzies over food. Hey it happens to the best of us. Food is instant gratification our clutch player when we feel the need to pacify ourselves. Food never says NO!!!!!!! Never disappoints us. Never hurts our feelings. Never abandons us. Our worries disappear for a moment when we munch on those fries or those tasty cupcakes or whatever comfort food brings you delight. Those are just a few of my weaknesses. We step on the scale and suddenly food was our silent frenemy. We feel betrayed. Hay food I loved you and this is how you pay me back in pounds (smile). Food can be your best friend or your worst enemy. You must set boundaries with your food relationship and deal with food accordingly just like any other relationship in your life.

Our relationship with food not only affects our life it also is an indication of our self-control, self-discipline, self-worth, self-love and reflects our self-sabotaging ways. Does this make any sense? Most of us would not allow people to betray our trust and take advantage of us or allow people in our lives who we knowingly do not have our best interest at heart. Yet when it comes to eating we allow food to overstep its boundaries and walk all over us and betray our healthy eating habits. This becomes your health blueprint. So do we blame the food or do we blame ourselves? Most will never shoulder the blame of becoming overweight and unhealthy. They will fault everyone else for their lack of self-control. They will say: "It's their fault for offering me a slice of pie to begin with". They rationalize and tell themselves if the fast food place was not on the way home they would have never stopped at the drive-thru. Wait, they even justify their lack of self-control and discipline and blame the supermarkets for putting those dozen of cookies on sale right when they started clean eating. I have to really extend you tough love in these instances. It is your fault!

Ok I said it! Learn your triggers and hot buttons that cause you to abandon your health goals. Ok let's get back to strategizing and transitioning you from selecting poor food choices to eating healthier more well-balanced planned meals.

Learning what foods are health friendly and knowing which foods to stay away from, affords you an opportunity to create a strategy in gaining back your control over your health and body which ultimately transforms into a healthy inspired way of living.

The proper food supplies our bodies our nutritional needs for energy production. Food fuels our body in order to perform and live at our most optimal levels. Foods either assist our body in aging gracefully or they work against us causing our bodies to age prematurely. You should be shopping and selecting foods from the perimeter aisles of the grocery store which is a great strategy for staying the course and sticking to healthy food choices. The foods located in the center aisles are typically processed, refined manufactured foods loaded with saturated fats, sodium, refined sugars, preservatives and fillers that are unhealthy. By shopping the outside aisles you won't pass by the good food choices up, this will ensure you do not bring those frenemies home. Everybody has opened their refrigerator or pantry and thought where did all this junk food come from? Well it did not invite itself you sent that invitation and the food shows up with a plus one. Going grocery shopping can be tricky. Many people rush out and go unprepared aimlessly walking the aisles and selecting items randomly. Another good idea is to never venture out to the grocery store on an empty stomach. An empty stomach sends the wrong ques and signals to your brain. You add extra burden to your will power on an empty stomach you are more prone to pick up that pizza, ice cream, soda, cookies and more likely to select foods for snacking versus whole food choices. So our main objective is going to the grocery store prepared with a list in hand on a mission. It is important not only to have the right foods on your grocery list but your list serves as the mission plan because it is very easy to jump ship and abort well meaningful intentions. Having the best intentions in the world means nothing if the proper foods don't make it home with you. Plan ahead, write it down so it will be plain and in sight and properly executed.

Get In Tuned.........Stay In Tuned

Getting in tuned with yourself allows you to see the beauty of your own reflection in the mirror. Often times we tend to compare ourselves to others, comparison robs us of the beauty of our uniqueness and leaves our mind with feelings of unworthiness and inadequacy. The good old apples to oranges comparison syndrome of course we all have been guilty of the comparison game a time or two, three, four or more. Comparison comes from a deep seated feeling that we do not measure up in life. The beautiful woman on the beach with the perfect hour glass figure, the coworker who has had children and snapped back to her pre-pregnancy weight, your friend who seems to have all her ducks in a row, the stranger in the grocery store who appears perfect, the woman at the gym with the great physique, women are more prone to compare their self, their life and of course their bodies to other women. The first rule of thumb in feeling great about yourself is to know who you are. When you are confident and know who you are you will never feel compelled to compare yourself to anyone in life. Know that you are the only YOU that exist in life. There are no two people that are the same in this world and that even goes for twins. What works for one person may not work for you and vice versa. If your journey looks totally different that is because we all are uniquely created differently.

God may have created all men equal but we surely are different down to our DNA. Take two women who are the exact same age, same weight, same height yet their bodies do not look the same due in part to genetics, body type, body shape and lifestyle. Not to mention even twins can't be compared to one another, sure they may look a whole lot alike but down to their DNA they are different. We really have to master this lesson on the comparison game. Once you have learned to live a life of no comparisons, your life will open up and create more space and time to love who you are from the inside out. Live a NO Comparisons Life!!!!!!

Let's focus on YOU right now. Yes You!!!!! Do you know what the statistics are for each and every human that makes it from conception to birth? You are SPECIAL!!!!!!! One of a KIND ORIGINAL.!!!!!!! That alone should be cause for you to stretch out your arms and hug yourself and declare: "I AM SPECIAL! I AM MADE IN GOD'S IMAGE".

Warning!!!...This is a very powerful affirmation, if you believe it, speak it you will reap all the benefits of this declaration in due time. Say it over and over and over and over repetitiously. Whenever you doubt your ability, or feeling like you do not measure up repeat positive affirmations over yourself daily. Being positive and optimistic about your life is the foundation of fertile imagery allowing you to grow into your best version of what God planned and designed you to be in this world.

We sometimes make the mistake of getting so overly caught up in our physical looks and the looks of others that we dismiss all other redeeming characteristics that make us unique and beautiful. Women will define and attach their worth to their physical attributes and body measurements. Being physically attractive for many women has become their only goal in life. Sure we all want to look our best that is not where the problem lies. Focusing totally on the physical becomes problematic and creates the snowball rolling down the hill of misplaced feelings about our self-worth. Trying to keep up appearances at the expense of our entire well-being affects our health in the long run. Looking good on the outside does not always correspond to feeling good and healthy on the inside.

It is very important we feel worthy and deserving and feel beautiful no matter what society says, or that magazine displays, or anybody's opinion on the subject. When we feel great about ourselves it reveals beauty irrespective to age, color, size, height, weight, physical appearances by anybody's limited standards.

We grow up hearing you are built or shaped just like your mother or your father or some family member near and dear to you or hey maybe far and not so dear. This may be good for some maybe not so good for others. Well the cold hard truth is drum roll please........our body type and shape have been handed down via genetics which we know life and genetics does not play fair. Sometimes genetics gives us great attributes then there are times genetics slaps our hand with a No-No and says: "I did not say you can eat that" (laugh out loud).

Let's now talk about the different body types that we all tend to fall into with some overlapping. Have you ever heard people describe another person being a bird and being able to eat anything they desire? On the other side of the spectrum you hear people talk about how if they even so much as glance at food they will gain weight without a mere bite. Ha! There is some validity to these claims on how our bodies metabolize foods and how our body gains weight and loses it. And it really has to do with body type, metabolism and genetics and the food we eat.

Below are the 3 general body types. All body types should consume the most natural sources of protein, healthy carbs and good essential fats. However, the daily caloric intake and exercise regimen should be tailored respective to the following body types.

- **Ectomorph Body Type:** Naturally slender build, hard weight gainers, typically can eat anything they want without consequences of weight gain.
- **Mesomorph Body Type:** Muscular build, body responds fast to exercise and lean muscle gains,

fast quick firing metabolism, very lean defined core
(ab formation).

- **Endomorph Body Type:** Body tends to gain
  weight easy, sluggish metabolism, stores fat easy
  over entire body, body does not quickly respond
  to regular exercise and requires strict diet
  regimen.

Your body type does not mean you can't reach your
fitness and health goals. However, knowing how your
body metabolizes food and responds to weight gain or
weight loss can be very beneficial in accessing your
overall health blueprint. When you understand certain
dynamics of health and fitness it allows you to customize
a strategic personal plan to be successful on your health
and wellness journey. Many complain that they never see
their results because they have not factored in specific
variables that affect their weight loss. There is not a one
size fits all diet or exercise regimen.

Chapter 4

Ageless Spirit Young At Heart

Fiercely Protect Your Inner Child......Stay Young at Heart, Mind, Body and Soul......

Maintaining a youthful outlook primarily originates in our brain whereby the brain sends out positive signals to our entire body that aligns with the originating thought. If our mind holds the belief that age is a hindrance, the body will align with these negative thoughts of this seed that is planted. So it is vitally important to feed and plant positive affirmations in your mind's soil. The mind is very moist and absorbent it is fertile ground. The mind is always open and receptive to prosperous thoughts or the mind is open to lack, poverty and unhealthy habits in every aspect of our lives. We are in constant struggle with our mind, thoughts and what we see manifest in our lives. Always stay young at heart and guard your childlike thirst for learning and growing. Remember To Stay Positive Always!!

As children we are encouraged by our parents, family and teachers to dream big and set goals, learn the ropes and do the best we can. As adults all these things become child's play and we quickly lose our zest for living an inspired life. We may have followed goals or aspirations other than our own choosing that has led us to unfulfilling accomplishments in our lives. You may have gotten so far down the path you feel there is no way to turn back now. No matter how far you have journeyed down a different path, I will not venture to say wrong because every path is meant to teach us something in life. No matter if you are at the beginning, in the middle or the end of this path, there is always time to start a new journey in life. You are only charged with living out your full expression in life, no matter how much you feel you missed the window of opportunity. I want to dispel all negative expressions that keep you from moving forward. Windows of opportunity do not exist with God.

This is God's universe he does not need a window, phone, door or any person place or thing to bless you with what he has ordained over your life. All that exist is your mind, your belief and faith in knowing that your thoughts, words line up with what you practice daily. Living life through our fullest expression activates endorphins and keeps our bodies vibrating at a certain frequency that maintains our youthfulness. When you live a fulfilling satisfying life your spirit is vibrating at very high frequencies. You radiate from the inside out because you are living out your God given purpose.

Fill your life with things that bring your heart joy and bring your mind peace. Many times we will get into a place of doing the popular thing to do. So we find ourselves being unpopular with our own joy. Society pushes us to go with the flow, follow the leader, or become the next carbon copy of someone else. In today's society we have become the ultimate click and follow culture. A world heavily influenced by social media norms, hashtags and status quos that leave individuality out of the equation. If everybody is doing it, then you should too, hurry up stand in the long line that manufactures massed produced lifestyles or surgery inspired bodies and the group think herd mentality. It is great to be inspired by the images and post of social media. The word needs all the inspiration it can get. But we have to keep our eyes open not to follow everything blindly and lose our own sense of self. Your sense of self is a valuable commodity in today's marketplace. Be careful not to lend this commodity to everybody else's bottom line. Ensure your thoughts, every word you speak and ultimately the way you feel about yourself is going into your personal account and strengthening your own portfolio. Always balance your ledger to reap your full benefits of your assets. Let go of other's opinions and hang ups and limited views those are liabilities you can't afford to maintain. Cut your losses and stay in the black.

We all are purposed in this LIFE! Have you ever noticed when you are doing something you love the time flies by, on the other hand when you are doing something you hate it becomes an arduous, tedious and cumbersome chore and the clock ticks by slowly. Ageless spirits follow their own unique paths and do not live in the anxiety of trying to fit in. Trust your intuition, your faith, your follow through and your purpose.

Get out of your head and move into your light. The light will guide you God shines the light on all of our footsteps whether the path goes off course. Many want to delete the footsteps they made in the dark seasons of their life. No God ordered your steps accordingly every step is blessed whether you feel it is or not. Every foot step you make leads you to your ultimate purpose. Life is the ultimate FITBIT app. In the end all of our steps add up and count as BLESSED!

Chapter 5

Body Image
The Beauty of Confidence

Confidence is the Most Ideal Body Type That Is not Reflected in Pounds on a Scale.........

Studies have shown that many women have suffered from some sort of body image issue(s) in their lifetime. As women we are unfairly judged on our looks and how we stack up to other women. Women size each other up. When we don't look like the models in the magazines, we beat ourselves up and slowly become the enemy within. Some become overly obsessed chasing a body image if it kills them and in some cases it literally does. Body issues believe it or not, often unknowingly impact many other areas in our lives. Those feelings of unworthiness or not being good enough creep into our minds and become weeds that sprout and drown out our positive thinking. Our mindset is essential to thrive and live in abundance here on earth. Working on our mind and gaining confidence, gives us inner strength and the power we need to deal with all of the outside distractions and media images that bombard us daily outlining society's ideal of standard beauty. There is no shortage of barely 20 something year olds (maybe younger) beautiful young slender physically fit women advertising and promoting every product under the sun and subliminally tapping into the subconscious minds of many. Those unrealistic and false images do not reflect all women, we all should feel beautiful for who we are. Your beauty within is much more significant than your age, height, size, color, shape. Body size and shape and labels have no place or space in true health and wellness. We all need a good dose of Vitamin "ME" which translates to loving "YOU". Ensuring you have positive thoughts and declaring affirmations over yourself builds your confidence and self-esteem to operate in your higher purpose of being.

Confidence is the invisible beauty that others see that has nothing to do with the physical but it is our beauty expressed via internal love for ourselves. The facade of the body and what people can see is more about what other's perceptions and views are of us which are limited by their eyesight. The view we hold of ourselves is a very powerful tool in connecting with the world and is far more important than anyone's opinion.

There are many times we are not feeling as confident as we would like which is normal we all have been there before. Have you ever walked into a room full of people and instantly felt you wanted to walk right back out of the door because maybe you felt you were underdressed or overdressed or felt insecure in some way? Socializing can become a bit of a challenge when we hold negative images of what we think people are saying behind our backs or whispering in their hidden thought bubbles. We get up in our own heads and make up versions of conversations of how we think people feel about us. Our self-confidence or lack thereof can hold us back or it can propel us forward in life. We all need a boost of self-confidence from time to time.

Even people who we assume have all the self confidence in the world. There is not a soul on earth who has never had to work on feeling more confident in some area in their lives. Once you master your self-confidence you will start to eliminate those anxiety feelings and gain confidence rooted in self-awareness and perfect the abilities to create a life full of enjoyment.

Chapter 6

Mindset Wellness

Transform Your Mind...... Transform Your Life.........
The mind is our biggest resistance to our optimal health and wellness
if you allow it to be. So make your mind your most powerful
alliance.......

There are gyms and fitness centers where we can go to
exercise and work on our physical body. We will
purchase a gym membership which is wonderful, as we
should see the importance of working on our temple it is
our residence in this life. However, there is not a brick
and mortar gym to exercise our mind. Let me take that
back we do have the library which we could technically
consider a gym for the mind right? Mindset health always
gets overlooked on many health journeys. Health and
wellness cannot exist without the mind. Many will stop
their health and wellness plan when they do not see
immediate results. They will say: "Oh it's simply not
working for me, I haven't lost an inch". Then go right
back to their comfort zone of emotional eating and a

sedentary lifestyle. We all have fallen off the wagon from time to time that is not the deal breaker. The deal breaker is underestimating how much your mind is in control. The mind is the prevailing muscle over all muscles in the body. If you do not exercise your mind there is no way to transform your body, your life, your dreams, your reality and everything else worth having in this life. Can you be healthy and not go to the gym? Sure you can but you can never be completely healthy without full control over your mindset. Solving your health issues without your mind will never work. Grant it you may have some success with reaching a few goals but it never fails you will always succumb to some underlying pattern of weakness in your mind waiting to trip you up again. When your equation factors the unknown variable (M) which is equal to mindset only then can you resolve to solve your health and wellness.

As I mentioned earlier many of us concentrate more on the outward appearance of others as well as ourselves. We enjoy looking great in our clothes and receiving compliments on how nicely dressed, color coordinated, accessorized and put together we appear to be. Yes I believe we all should put our best foot forward when we step out of the confines of our home into the world. As I subscribe to the saying "You never get a 2nd chance to make a 1st impression". However, adorning your body with clothes, shoes and jewelry will never substitute for a healthy body and a life of longevity. A healthy conditioned body looks good in anything and better naked. There are people who would not think twice on the price tag of clothing but find it fruitless to invest in their health and wellness. It is not important how great you look in your clothes when your body is in an unhealthy state. The thought that you can fake real health with the best wardrobe reflects a faulty mindset blueprint. In order for our body to be in complete balance, our mind and spirit should also be exercised. At the very crux of optimal health and wellness is a healthy mind. We don't look at exercising our mind or the importance of brain health when thinking overall health and fitness. Consider the mind our Central Processing Unit (CPU) our bodies do not work without the function of our mental faculties. The brain sends instructions on how the body should work. If you lift your arm over your head, bend down to pick up something, yawn, walk, run, talk, think, feel all the way down to our reasoning abilities our brain has to send signals to our body parts to complete these task. So it's clear to see who really is in charge of our lives. Our mind lets us know daily who the big boss is. However, we employ our mind which makes us technically in charge of the corporation and our mind is our actual employee that works on behalf of our corporation.

The expression mind over matter pretty much describes the process of eating properly and exercising when we much rather be sprawled out on the couch relaxing watching our favorite TV show and crunching on those chips. Gaining control over our thoughts includes managing our emotions as it relates to the practice of conscientious eating habits. Mastering your thoughts, training your mind is the only way to overcome the bad habit of emotional eating. You are going to have to become keenly aware of your stress triggers sending you into the pleasure principle of eating. Healthy ageless people do not eat for pleasure or to make them feel good. Healthy people practice constructive eating habits. And you can too. Praying to God alone will not do it! God created us with everything we need to overcome every obstacle in our lives including our health, self-control over what we choose to think, believe and ultimately put in our bodies.

Your mind can work for you or against you in your quest for ultimate wellness. Let's now look at what we can do to keep the mind fit and in shape to help us reach our weight loss and health maintenance goals.

Make a habit of eating nutrient rich foods to support brain health. The following are foods we need to incorporate into our daily diets that greatly improve our brain's functions.

Your next trip to the farmer's market and/or your neighborhood grocery store should include picking some of these foods up and putting them on your menu today!

- **Blueberries:** Blueberries can be considered BRAINBERRIES. They hold the highest antioxidant level of all the fresh fruits, promotes hemoglobin and oxygen in the blood.

- **Wild Pink Salmon:** Wild Pink Salmon is packed with essential fatty acids Omega 3's, protein, vitamin D, niacin and selenium.

- **Nuts and Seeds:** The following nuts (walnuts, hazelnuts, brazil nuts, almonds, cashews, peanuts, sunflower seeds, sesame seeds, flax seed); offers an alternative source of protein, fiber and healthy fats.

- **Avocados:** Avocados are fatty fruit loaded with unsaturated good fats and vitamin E, helps the body absorb fat soluble vitamins A, D, and K.

- **Freshly brewed teas:** The following teas: (Green tea, Black tea, White Tea, Red tea, Grey Tea): Tea also has potent antioxidants, especially the class known as catechins. Catechins are specifically a part of the (flaven-3-ol) of natural phenol and antioxidant, which promotes healthy blood flow.

- **Broccoli and Cauliflower:** Broccoli and cauliflower are good sources of choline and vitamin B known for its role in brain development.

Chapter 7

Poor Health and Sedentary Lifestyle

Don't Feed Me Grapes......I Will Pick Them from the Vine and Stomp them into Wine..... There is no Luxury in Laziness..........

As we discussed earlier gravity has its place with aging but, poor health not only takes a front seat it accelerates aging by stepping on the gas pedal. When we are battling poor health due to poor eating and a sedentary lifestyle it robs us from living life as God designed. God intricately designed our bodies to be strong yet delicate with resilience and to heal from the inside out. Food gives our bodies energy to live, heal and recover by providing our body the required nutrients. The healthier the food source, the more effective and efficient our body works.

If the body is not fed the proper foods it starts to weaken over time every cell and organ in our body requires quality nutrition from food, water and supplementation where appropriate. When we eat the wrong foods our body's eco-system become out of alignment which onsets many health issues.

Poor nutrition compounded with not moving our bodies enough to burn the calories we consume daily leads to weight gain which leads to poor health. What we consume activates good health or accelerates bad health. The USA has one of the highest rates of obesity in the world we have become the super-sized fast food and processed western society. We are the hurry up make it fast in a jiffy better known as the microwavable culture. We don't have time to prepare our meals, we don't have time to sleep, and we don't have time to spare to workout. By now, we should all know that poor nutrition leads to the following health conditions:

- High Blood Pressure
- Diabetes
- High cholesterol
- Over weight
- Immobility
- Heart disease
- Cardiovascular disease
- Intestinal problems

- Colon cancer
- Liver disease
- Kidney malfunction
- Death

There is so much to be said about eating healthy. Eating a well-balanced diet and exercising regularly along with keeping our emotions and stress in control can help us combat and prevent many health issues and diseases of the body to live out a long fruitful life.

There are two variables that rob us faster of our youth which are poor health and a sedentary lifestyle. Life has become fast paced where we tend to cut corners and want satisfaction and gratification now. We eat on the go, we are not active on a daily basis, we enjoy eating while lying down watching television or even reading a book for hours. We must take the elevator versus the stairs. We park our cars as close to our destination even if it means throwing our hazard lights and double parking because it's an emergency to get in and out quick. You will also see people drive in circles and wait on a parking space to try and circumvent walking a few extra steps, they will boldly say "that's way too much walking for me".

It is this mentality that keeps people from getting the best out of life through our daily active routines. When we are not active and sit for long periods of time on end, it is a precursor for poor health and kick starts the aging process. It is worthy to note that some individuals are dealing with genetic disorders and require special treatment and this will have a huge impact on one's aging process. For most of us we are healthy to a point we can control and maintain a healthy lifestyle through diet and exercise without medical intervention.

Americans are eating more and moving less. We live in a world that rewards laziness. A technology focused broken society seeking quick fixes, latest trends, yo-yo diets, teas, tonics big sigh. We have developed a preoccupation with perfecting the illusion of health. Women want the perfect hour glass figure but they do not want to invest in real health. They invest in hocus pocus and magic trick waist trainers that promise to decrease your waistline if worn every day for the rest of their lives. They are throwing money at the screen and squeezing a size 38" waist into a 26" waist trainer like WHALAAAAA. I am always amazed at the torture women are ready set willing to endure in the name of vanity and risky unhealthy ill-informed strategies that disregard true health. They will shun or avoid working out and eating healthy because they have told themselves it's too much hard work. No matter if their waist is bursting at the seams like a can of biscuits when the waist-trainer is taken off. When one product does not work they jump on to the next fly by night magic trick. Many women and men are at war with their bodies when in all actuality the battle field is in their mindset. They do not understand the importance of self-compassion and self-love and not hating your body to yield the long lasting results they seek. Hiding behind clothes and torture garments sweeps the real issue(s) under the carpet. When you address the core issue you are picking that carpet up and sweeping underneath it properly, so you don't continue to trip over and over again. Understanding it was neglect of loving thyself and taking good care of your health in the first place that created the ground swell or in this instance the bulging belly. You put your health off far too long you said: "You don't have the time, you will start next week, you don't have the money, you don't feel like eating healthy today, you don't feel like exercising after a long day at the office". Excuse after excuse and before you know it, your weight has tipped the scale to your dismay and surprise. What you put off today is waiting for you tomorrow and the next day and all days thereafter. You cannot ignore your health and wellness. It has a very unique way of catching up with you and demanding your attention. By the time it gets to that point you are suffering from health ailments then you guess maybe it's time to make a change. Your health is not any one's priority but your own. It's ok to seek the assistance of a personal trainer or nutritionist sure but they are not responsible for what you should be doing and that is taking care of your needs mentally, physically and spiritually. Personal trainers, health coaches and health mentors like myself provide excellent motivation and provide you with nutritional recommendations and exercise plans but you hold sole proprietorship of the health business of "YOU". We work for you! Not the other way around.

Let go of all the quick sells and promises that offer you the body of your dreams in an hour, a day or just a week without real work. Get rid of the mindset that you can take the shortcut or forgo the workouts to get that nice trim lean body, instead wake up to the body of your reality. Wake up make the decision the commitment to do what it takes to reach your goals daily. All goals are obtainable via a decision 1st, action plan 2nd, effort 3rd, and last but not least consistency. There is no way of getting around the work aspect of it all. Those who live great lives work at it. Those who live healthy and fit lives work at it. Those who reach their goals in life simply work at it. The satisfaction and fulfillment of working on yourself always pays you for the work you rendered. Would you pay someone that did not provide the work you hired them to do? Then why would the universe grant you anything worth having if you have not planted and cultivated the seeds. Just in case you did not know, you can't just plant the seeds and come back and expect a full garden. Your seeds require you to nurture, speak, water and pull the weeds in order to reap your harvest. You want real results those results are always found in real work.

We have adopted this mindset that sitting still and being inactive as a luxury of living THE GOOD LIFE! Many of us have careers that have enabled us to become more inactive throughout the day than 25 years ago. Our daily work includes sitting for long periods of time communicating or interacting with others globally without having to physically move a muscle. We are able to talk, type, text and skype for hours on end without getting up from our chairs. Some even find luxury in working from the comfort of their homes and boost about not even having to leave the bed in their pajamas. We sit and stare at the computer and phone screens all day which is a cause for concern for many who do not implement strategies to break the monotony of a sedentary life and work style. Sitting at the computer for hours with no breaks takes its toll on your health. There are certain health issues that arise from desk jobs most commonly carpel tunnel syndrome to varicose veins due to restricted blood circulation. If not properly addressed poor blood circulation can lead to more serious complications such as blood clots over time.

9 Quick Easy Ways to Combat Work Place Sedentary Habits

1) Stand up and stretch {5 - 10 mins for every hour you are sitting}.

2) Take frequent breaks that allow you to walk and get your blood circulating and flowing {walk to restroom even if you don't have to go}.

3) Make lunchtime an active FIT BREAK, take a 20 min brisk walk outside.

4) Walk up or down a couple of flights of stairs to keep the blood circulating.

5) Squeeze a stress ball throughout the day {improves blood flow}.

6) Stand up and sit down in chair repeat this exercise as needed.

7) Drink lots of water and fluids throughout the day to keep your system flushed and hydrated also gives you incentive to walk to the restroom {No sodas or heavily caffeinated drinks}.

8) Eat light healthy snacks to keep your energy up and stabilize blood sugar levels.

9) Raise your arms over your head, ball up your fist squeeze release {repeat as needed}.

Chapter *8*

Stress the Silent Culprit and Hidden Gotcha

Put Your Stress to Rest...... And Set Your Clock to Inspired Living.........

When our bodies get stressed it can produce every symptom in the book of illness. Stress weakens the body's immune system making our bodies susceptible to germs, viruses and sickness. Our bodies are designed to handle good and bad stress on a daily basis. Good stress is called **"Eustress"** where our bodies respond to what we perceive as favorable conditions like winning the lottery, graduating from college, passing your driver's exam, landing your dream job or getting married. Bad stress is called **"Distress"** when our bodies perceive fear, worry and or overload such as losing your job, involved in a car accident, envisioning a snake at your feet, fear of a plane crashing or a fear of heights. Distress can lead to various issues resulting in disease.

Stress can lead to high blood pressure, heart attacks, stomach and digestive issues, headaches, body tension, aches and never ending insomnia. The trite saying: "Our beauty lies in our rest", is a very true statement. Not getting enough quality sleep is sure to wreak havoc on not only our physical being but both emotionally and mentally. The word "STRESS" itself includes the Letters "REST".....AHA!

So you have gotten into a workout routine and eating healthier there's yet another variable tugging at your youth strings. Stress is a huge monumental factor when it comes to aging over the course of our lifetime. Our stress levels directly impact how we age. Learning to combat and manage stress is one way to slow down the hands on the clock of time.

Stress is the reason for an inordinate number of doctor's office visits each year. Stress combined with a poor diet and lack of exercise is a number one killer. It can increase the risk of heart attacks and strokes it can provoke and bring on just about every ailment imaginable. Disease starts when our cells are overwhelmed and maxed out when the cell is under attack. Our best defense against our bodies aging as a result of stress is rest, relaxation, prayer, positive thoughts and breathing techniques and eating a healthy diet to include adaptogens super powerful foods. You may have never heard of adaptogens and wondering what on earth are adatogens?

Adaptogens can be found in plant based whole foods as well as quality supplements. Adaptogens decrease our cellular sensitivity to stress in other words they internally help our body deal with bad stress favorably. Managing our stress triggers appropriately is the way we throw a life saver to consciously rescue our self. Learning your stress cues and responding in a positive and favorable manner will improve the quality of your day and extend your lifespan.

Start to become more aware of your stress triggers. Listen to your body's ques that signal you to slow down and RESET. When you start to feel overwhelmed take a Deep Breath Close Your Eyes and RELAX.

Chapter 9

Breathe In Life

A Breath of Air is Life Itself.....Energy to the Soul.....

Breathing is our life source! A newborn baby takes their very first breath, which simultaneously starts both the lifecycle and aging process. One of the very first things we are advised to do in any situation or circumstance if we are panicked or traumatized is to TAKE A DEEP BREATH. For instance, the mother in labor is reminded to breathe in deep through the nostrils and blow out slowly through the mouth to relax the body and dull the pain of the birthing process. The yoga coach gently reminds you to breathe and remember your mantras bringing the mind back in focus so the body can relax comfortably into challenging yoga positions. When we are overly excited or extremely upset taking a deep breath relaxes our body to combat the stress that is attacking our body's internal defense system. The novice competitor or people new to health and fitness will underestimate or even trivialize proper breathing techniques. People who are well seasoned in fitness and training or competing in extremely higher performance echelons where the body is challenged physically for long periods of time are fully conscious and well adapted to proper breathing techniques.

You are at your Doctor's office and the first request is to take a deep breath in while he places the stethoscope on your chest and back. The Doctor is listening for any indications of obstruction to your air pathways as well as fluid in the lungs. Assessing the health of your lungs is crucial to our entire body. The lungs are not considered a muscle, but our lungs need to be healthy and strong. The lungs provide the entire body its oxygen source while removing carbon dioxide from the body. We are able to go days without eating and drinking however, we are unable to go seconds without oxygen and air flow without damaging major organs like our brain. When the body has been deprived of oxygen our brain shuts down rendering our whole entire body useless.

Now let's talk a little more about the benefits of deep breathing and how it can preserve your overall health resulting in a more youthful glow from destressing. Our lungs have the capacity to hold up to 6 liters of air and most of us spend our time on this earth shallow breathing. There are many benefits to incorporating daily deep breathing exercises to your healthy living blueprint.

- **Breathing detoxifies:** Our body is designed to release 70% of its toxins through breathing. When you exhale from the body you are releasing the carbon dioxide that passes through your bloodstream into your lungs.
- **Breathing releases tension:** The body's response to fear, anger, stress and tension has a very negative impact on our bodies. It constricts our muscles, blood vessels and places stress on our hearts and brains. When we are tense our breathing becomes shallow and does not allow proper oxygen flow to our cells.
- **Breathing relaxes the mind/body and brings clarity:** Oxygenation of the brain reduces

excessive anxiety levels and puts the body in a relaxed state.

- **Breathing increases digestion and assimilation of food:** Proper breathing improves our digestive organs such as the stomach. When the stomach receives proper amounts of oxygen the digestion process is enhanced and your body digests food more effective and efficiently.

- **Breathing improves the nervous system:** The brain, spinal cord and nerves receive increased oxygen as a result the whole body is more nourished.

- **Breathing assists in weight control:** The extra oxygen burns up excessive fat more efficiently. And vice versa if you are underweight the oxygen feeds the starving tissues and glands.

- **Breathing enhances your mood:** Proper breathing increases the pleasure inducing neurochemicals in the brain to elevate your mood and combat physical pain.

So with all these great benefits to breathing by now you are ready to start breathing life and vitality into your body. In order to breathe properly and get the oxygen flowing you need to breathe deeply into your abdomen not just your chest. A critical part to breathing is regulating your breaths 3 to 5 seconds IN.....and 3 to 5 seconds OUT.

If possible go to a nice quiet relaxing place, or quiet room in your home/workplace or maybe a park to reap the full benefits of deep breathing exercises. These deep breathing exercises can be done with visualization for maximum results. When visualizing with deep breathing focus and concentrate on positive images and hold the thought for at least 10 secs. Imagine yourself....
HAPPY, HEALTHY and WEALTHY!!!

You want to inhale through your nose, expanding your belly, and expanding your chest. Hold for 5 seconds. Exhale fully with a slightly parted mouth, blow out until lungs are completely empty (repeat as needed).

Chapter 10

Beautiful Foods Yield a Younger You

Eat Beautiful Foods.....Drink More H2O.......

This may sound like another trite recommendation but it has been proven that when we consume more natural whole foods, fruits and veggies it maintains our body's pH level. When the body becomes too acidic we develop chronic illness(s) and it also makes us age quickly. There are three beliefs that govern and form most of our lives. You Are What You THINK! You Are What You SPEAK! And last but not least You Are What you EAT! More than likely you have heard them all before. During our younger years we were not too concerned about what we thought, spoke and ate. Aging, health and wellness pretty much was not at the forefront or a high priority. Growing older typically pulls the carpet out from underneath our feet when we hit our 40's. The 40's seems to be the multiple where we start to rearrange and change our priorities with respect to our health. Typically a lot of people may have experienced or are dealing with some sort of health issue that requires their immediate attention.

This is their wake up call to action where they usually start to watch what they eat and implement an exercise program. In your 40's you can start to lose some of your energy levels due to the fact the body slows its production of many essential vitamins such as vitamin B-12 and hormone production. Over the years the 40's had been considered and deemed middle age before the millennium era. People are living healthier and longer pushing the median lifespan past the 40's. In the new millennium the 40's are not so much middle age, but rather the multiple where we come into an awaking of self-awareness. We have lived 4 decades of our lifetime and by 40 we should be wiser but the 40's does not come without its fair share of health and body challenges. During our 40's we notice that our metabolism does not fire up as fast as it did 2 decades ago. We long for our teenage years and the twenties where we could eat without cause for concern of impending weight gain. We realize now we have to work harder and smarter to ensure our bodies are functioning and hitting on all cylinders as we age. Many foods are praised for their amazing abilities to preserve our youthful appearance and assist in supplementing many of the nutrients our bodies lose due to aging. You will be surprised at which foods hail as miracle foods you may have been eating them all along.

Antioxidants

Antioxidants can be found naturally in plant-based foods such as fruits, vegetables, coffee, tea, wine, and even dark chocolate. While there are thousands of antioxidant compounds out there, you've probably heard of flavanols (found in chocolate), resveratrol (found in wine), and lycopene (found in tomatoes). Other popular antioxidants include vitamins A beta carotene, C, E, and catechins.

Foods high in antioxidants when consumed transfer their healing properties to our cells, which helps to slow down the aging process and even reversing some damage due to poor health. Oxidation is a normal chemical reaction that occurs when free radicals form within the nucleus of our cells. This process is similar to what happens during the browning of an apple after it is sliced open and exposed to the oxygen in the air. The oxygen atoms in the air interact with the sugar in the apple, forming oxygen radicals. These radicals break down the flesh of the apple called oxidation and the apple begins to rot due to the enzymatic browning process.

Eat More Of The Following:

Watermelon

Lycopene is an antioxidant that gives watermelon and tomatoes their bright deep red color. It helps skin stave off UV damage, provides muscle and nerve support, It is an antioxidant and forms alkalinity in the body.

Pomegranates

The seeds of pomegranates are loaded with vitamin C and anthocyanins. Preventing fine lines, wrinkles and dryness and increasing collagen production which gives the skin a firmer look.

Blueberries

Blueberries supply the skin with vitamins C and E that work together to tighten and brighten skin. In addition, blueberries contain "Arbutin" a natural derivative of skin brightener "Hydroquinone".

Lobster

You will be very surprised to know that lobster is very high in zinc. As a matter of fact shellfish has anti-inflammatory properties that help treat a number of skin issues such as acne. Lobster is very high in essential fatty acids omega 3's, low in cholesterol, and great source of B12 and phosphorus.

Kale

Kale is packed with vitamin K and loads of iron. Vitamin K is known for its ability to promote healthy blood clotting. Very beneficial in preventing the blood vessels around the eyes from leaking which is known to cause the dark shading around the eyes. Yes the raccoon eye factor.

Walnuts

If walnuts were not already yummy enough the fact that they are very high in omega-3 fatty acids, vitamin E and copper, gives you even more reasons to enjoy. The Omega-3's help to keep the hair hydrated and nourished, while vitamin E helps maintain and repair damaged hair follicles. Walnuts also are high in copper the element that helps prevent the hair from graying.

Avocados

Packed with Omega-9 fatty acids, along with oleic acid helps keeps the outer layer of the skin's moisture content, makes the skin plump and supple, avocados are a very good source of healthy fats that are required in our diet.

Cantaloupe

Cantaloupe is just one of those fruits that's so tasty who cares about the benefits right? Well just in case you are inclined to know, this sweet melon contains beta carotene also known as vitamin A which regulates the skin's ability to rejuvenate while keeping the pores healthy and clear.

Prebiotics and Probiotics

We all have needed a dose of antibiotics a time or two in our lives. We need probiotics (strands of healthy bacteria) in our systems at all times. Probiotics is the good bacteria needed to maintain a healthy gut, colon and stools. Probiotics fight to keep our youth and beauty by reducing inflammation at a cellular level. There is one tricky aspect of probiotics they are delicate and once they enter your system the heat and stomach acid can render useless. To the rescue comes the Prebiotic.

A **Prebiotic** is a specialized plant fiber that nourishes the existing good bacteria in the large bowel or colon. Probiotics introduce the good bacteria into our gut, but prebiotics act as a fertilizer for the good bacteria that is already present in your system. Prebiotics support and help good bacteria grow and flourish. It improves the ratio of the good versus bad bacteria. This ratio has been proven to have a direct correlation to your overall health and wellbeing, from your stomach to the brain. The body does not digest the prebiotic plant fibers it in turns, provide many digestive and general health benefits to the entire body.

Green Tea

You may not be partial to teas. I am a tea versus everything else kinda girl. But after reading the benefits of green tea you may even develop an instant tea fetish yourself. Green tea is known for its high antioxidant levels. This tea contains high amounts of catechins these compounds can shield you from carcinogens which are known to cause cancer. Green tea also helps to lower bad cholesterol and is beneficial in the management of weight loss. So sip yourself to a healthy leaner you with green tea.

You should be standing in line at the grocery store by now after learning all the amazing benefits of antioxidants. Filler up with the aforementioned and immediately start reaping the benefits of a healthier beautiful you.

Chapter 11

Face Yoga: Smiling is Exercise

A Smile is Nature's Face Lift (Flex your facial muscles).......

Create a loving filled life where you have many opportunities and reasons to enjoy life and smile. Stop whatever you are doing, wherever you are and SMILE right now from ear to ear. You just increased your lifespan a few minutes so every time you smile you are adding additional minutes to your life. It is said people who smile often live longer lives. When you smile, you not only exercise certain muscles in your face which not only physically lifts the face and brightens your facial appearance but you evoke endorphins, an immediate mood enhancer without drugs or invasive plastic surgery. Studies have suggested a strong link between longevity and smiling. Smiling has been known to boost the immune system, lower blood pressure and promotes longevity.

Gravity takes such a huge toll on our facial features so when we smile it fights the good fight against the gravity pull on our face. In addition, smiling increases our endorphins, oxytocin, serotonin and can act as a natural pain killer. Smiling makes you look up to 3 years younger than a relaxed face or frowning. There are many health benefits to smiling:

- Instant mood enhancer
- Makes you look younger and more attractive
- Relieves stress
- Boost immunity
- Lowers blood pressure
- Natural face lift
- Evokes endorphins
- Increases longevity
- Improves self-confidence

So we see how smiling can instantly improve your quality of life and well-being if coupled with laughter it doubles the endorphins. It's also important to take care of your gums and teeth and practice good oral hygiene. The gums, tongue, teeth can be an indication of certain underlying health issues. Keeping your annual teeth cleaning appointment and following up on any outstanding dental work benefits not only your smile but your overall health. Never ignore a tooth ache seek medical assistance to properly treat tooth aches to prevent the infection from spreading to other critical areas of the body.

Tips on how to naturally brighten your smile instantly:

- Add a pinch of turmeric, baking soda and coconut oil when brushing
- Eat strawberries
- Drink lemon water
- Eat an apple a day
- Floss after meals
- Eat carrots and celery
- Wear darker or very bright lip color
- Get your annual teeth cleaning
- Oil Pulling

And while you are smiling do not neglect your lips. The skin on our lips is very delicate and needs moisture and protection every day. Be sure to keep your lips moisturized and protected with a SPF 30+ sunscreen.

Chapter 12

Acidity .vs. Alkalinity

And The Winner Is By an Unanimous Decision
An Alkaline Body Wins Every Fight!.........

The foods we eat can age us past our chronological birth age. Foods will either protect our cells and organs or they will attack and destroy them. The body should be in a positive pH state to maintain our body's healthy ecosystem. The body's pH level ranges from 0 - 14. A zero pH level is the peak of acidity; seven equals a neutral alkalinity; and fourteen equals optimal alkalinity. So what does the abbreviation pH stand for? The letters pH stand for "Potential of Hydrogen" in the body. All of our body's systems have a pH level from our blood, digestive tract to including our saliva. Health and wellness addresses the body's acidity state. It is a lifestyle that seeks to maintain our body's normal pH levels. So most will only focus on portion size which we should be mindful not to overeat but, the larger issue is the quality of our food sources to improve the body's alkaline state.

Eating a high alkaline diet helps the body reduce our daily acid load. The American diet primarily comprises of red meat, dairy, wheat, gluten, refined sugars, processed and fast foods. You may be asking the question "What are some alkaline food sources?" Great question! Any food or drink that promotes alkalinity in the body when eaten such as fruits (citrus), vegetables, spices and alkaline ionized water.

It is good to note the body is capable of maintaining an acid/alkaline balance on its own. However, certain food choices leave the body defenses slow and unresponsive which throws the body in a high acidity state. Therefore, the need to eat foods with high alkaline properties will always exist.

A fast easy safe way to immediately start your body's alkaline process is to eat raw, unprocessed natural foods to include fruits, vegetables and whole grains along with certain spices and healing teas. Below list some foods that aid in the alkaline process of the body.

Alkalizing Vegetables

- Beets
- Broccoli
- Cauliflower
- Celery
- Cucumber
- Kale
- Lettuce
- Onions
- Peas
- Peppers
- Spinach

Alkalizing Fruits

- Apples
- Bananas
- Berries
- Cantaloupe
- Grapes
- Melons
- Lemons
- Oranges
- Peaches

- Pears
- Watermelon

Alkalizing Protein

- Almonds
- Chestnuts
- Tofu

Alkalizing Spices

- Cinnamon
- Curry
- Ginger
- Mustard
- Sea Salt

Alkalizing Teas

- Yerba Mate tea
- Peppermint tea
- Ginger tea
- Rosemary tea
- Lavender tea
- Rosehip tea

Chapter 13

The Majestic Purple Food Power

Just Color Me Purple...... That Will Be Just GRAPE with Me......

We all know by now eating healthy means eating more foods with deep vibrant color. We pretty much have heard about the reds, the yellows, the browns, the oranges, the blues, the greens....but there is less mention of the purples.

Purple just happens to be one of my favorite colors so the fact that purple foods offer some of the highest levels of antioxidants makes sense as to why I absolutely love the color purple. So why does purple fruit and vegetables have the highest antioxidant concentration levels compared to all the other colors of fruits and vegetables? It's all in the color, the deepest darker color food provides higher benefits to our body. Purple foods are rich in anthocyanins and antioxidants and have been known to fight cancer and repair cell damage.

Below are some purple foods along with their health benefits that you should start including in your daily diet if you have not already:

- **Purple Onions** - Fights regenerative diseases and fungi, best source of quercetin, a bioflavonoid that has been found to scavenge free radicals in the body, anti-bacterial and anti-inflammatory properties, and has shown promising potential for preventing and controlling the formation of polyps, treating psoriasis and reducing the risk of stomach cancer.

- **Purple Grapes** - Very high in resveratrol which improves cardiovascular health, good source of fiber, lowers bad cholesterol levels, full of malic acid that assist in energy production to revitalize and repair damaged cells, contains lignans that help prevent breast cancer, contains oils that act as a potent natural antibiotic and improves the skin and structure of the veins.

- **Purple Cabbage** - Aids in digestion and is a blood builder, rich in minerals (calcium, potassium, choline, iodine, and sulphur), purple cabbage is an alkaline food that helps to regulate and balance our system. It also improves the brain functionality.

- **Purple Berries** - (Acai berries, Black berries, Elderberries, Black Currant berries and Chokeberries) – Extremely high in anthocyanins super powerful antioxidant, reduces inflammation in the body and destroys free radicals, high in fiber and improves bone health.

- **Purple Rice** - Purple Rice (Forbidden Royalty Purple Rice). This rice was once only reserved for royal and elite. Purple rice is unique in the fact that is bypasses the digestion process and directly feeds the body's cells with amino acids and polysaccharide peptides. This allows our cells to make and transport energy more efficiently.

- **Purple Egg Plants** - Egg Plants pack a very powerful purple punch of phenolic antioxidant compounds and "Nasunin". Nasunin is a heavy hitter free radical scavenger fighter known to protect lipids (fats) in our brain cells that keeps our brain healthy. Egg Plants help improve cardiovascular health and lowers bad cholesterol.

- **Purple Carrots** - It does not get any better than Purple carrots. Filled to the max with Beta carotene. Contains anthocyanins and antioxidants that preserve our youth factor. The blue purple pigment can enhance vision and improve memory, also promotes healthy heart and even supports weight control.

Chapter 14

Sleeping Beauty

The Age Old Adage....."Get Your Beauty Rest! Has profound significance especially in today's technology driven world that demands so much of our time, attention and resources......

You need to log out of all social media and online applications and be done with it all by a certain time each night. No sneak peeking to see your notifications. It can wait! Power the computer down, turn off all of your gadgets and precious devices. 30 years ago we were not checking our phones while lying in bed or working on the computer in the middle of the night. This has created bad sleeping habits for many. The fact that we are not getting a good night's sleep is compounded further with the disruption of artificial light known as "Blue Light". Our bodies have a natural circadian rhythm. Our circadian rhythm is our biological sleep clock that is driven on a 24 hour cycle that dictates our physiological processes. So have you ever notice you start to tucker out at a certain time each day? It is partly due to our circadian rhythms and our sleep/wake homeostasis patterns. So if we have been up for hours and burning the midnight oil our body starts to tell us we need to power down and recharge with sleep. When we don't get our required 8 hours of quality sleep it throws our bodies out of balance and off our natural body cycles.

Plan a nighttime routine that fosters relaxation to prime you for a quality night's rest. We prepare more for our morning routine, ensuring we eat a good breakfast, exercise, and shower to start the day. We go about our day in a planned manner meeting our goals and task on the day's agenda. However, our nightly rituals just turn out to be happenstance leaving everything up to chance. We allow ourselves to work into the wee-wee hours and eventually checking the time on the clock and saying "It's pretty late I better get some shut eye." By this time you only have 4-5 hours (even less) until the alarm clock or your phone chimes your favorite morning ringtone. Wake up! Wake up! Wake up! Time to make the donuts and in many cases eat them!

Sleeping is our body's restoration period where beautiful things happen. Things like healing, recovery, growth and rejuvenation and so much more. There are 5 Beauty rules that are required to maintain and preserve our youthfulness and sleep is in that top tier:

1) Beauty Rule #1   Natural Healthy Diet
2) Beauty Rule #2   Active Lifestyle
3) Beauty Rule #3   8 Hours Quality Sleep
4) Beauty Rule #4   Release Stress
5) Beauty Rule #5   Exercise Mind, Body and Spirit

We often downplay a good night's sleep. I hear so many people say "I don't need that much sleep" or "I can sleep when I am dead". Get out of the mindset that sleep is wasteful time that should be traded for working hours. Our mental and physical health requires a good quality rest period. Ever wake up feeling exhausted and at times more tired than when your head hits the pillow? Do you often toss and turn thinking about what you did not check off your "To Do List" and while lying in bed with your eyes closed creating an even longer "Extra To Do

List" in your mind's eye to accomplish the next day? Wishing you had more hours in your day to be productive to get more work done just so you can pile more work on your plate. We all know the negative effects of overloading our plate with way too much food does. But do we really stop to think about the negative impact of piling too many things "To Do" on our plate? The quality of your day, your sustained energy levels and mental clarity and focus depends on the body's resting phase. During the body's daily sleep phase, all of our organs, cells and systems are resetting. You may be thinking while your sleeping your body is sleeping along with you. In actuality our bodies are performing their nightly balance checks and refueling our body's functionality. So while we are off to "La La Dream Land" our brain is working the night shift doing clean up patrol on our waste removal function. Our brain executes these nightly checks when we reach our deepest level of the sleeping phase. This deep level of sleep is what is known as the REM sleep phase. Ever wonder how we are able to recall memories from our past?

Well while we are sleeping the brain is under construction working to cement all of our memories and thoughts from the day. Those memories include what is on your things to do list as well as our deeper thought processes and intellect.

Here are more reasons to fluff your pillow and create a nightly bedtime routine to foster quality sleep:

- **Improved Memory:** One of the things as we age that takes a hit is our memory. Affectionately known as our "Senior Moments". Our brain can start to lose those fast firing neurons that are required to learn new information, remember old information and our ability to focus as well as concentrate. Getting proper sleep enhances the brain functions and keeps the brain clear of brain fog and memory loss.

- **Live Longer:** Who would have thought getting our required sleep and napping to rest the entire body is linked to longevity? Hmmmmm... makes sense. No longer does sleep your life away apply, the old saying should be modified to read: "Sleep to add additional quality years to your life".

When the body is sleeping every organ, cell, system is allowed to regenerate and recover to work better during our waking hours.

- **Combats Inflammation:** Inflammation in the body can lead to heart disease, stroke, arthritis and premature aging. People who sleep six or fewer hours a night have higher blood levels of inflammatory proteins than people who get more hours of sleep. The C-reactive protein which is commonly associated with heart attack risk was higher in people who got fewer than 6 hours of sleep on a consistent basis.

- **Maintains Healthy Weight:** Yet another reason to say "Goodnight John Boy" a little earlier. People who are managing their weight through diet and exercise when well rested lose more fat than people who were sleep deprived, who lost more muscle mass. The body tends to feel hungrier when you're not properly rested. When you are sleepy certain hormones rise in your bloodstream these particular hormones drive the appetite. Sleep and metabolism are controlled by the same sectors of the brain.

- **Lowers Stress Levels**: Sleep and stress are very closely associated. Sleep deprivation has been link to many health issues and can be a huge risk in performing our daily routines. Certain mission critical jobs even require professionals to inform management if they are tired and unrested such as (pilots, police officers, truck drivers, emergency personnel and surgeons). As it can be a hazard to your job responsibilities and duties when sleep deprived. Getting a quality night sleep is critical for everyone to function at our highest performance level. Sleep can reduce our level of stress and controls factors such as blood pressure and cholesterol.

Chapter 15

Spice Up Your Life

Variety May Be the Spice of LIFE.....However Spice Itself Preserves LIFE!.......

Adding spices to your meals is a quick easy way to improve your current health. Who knew adding flavor to your favorite foods could ultimately improve and save your life so to speak. For centuries spices and herbs have been used by naturopathic healers to improve and even heal people of various health issues. Many over the counter traditional prescribed drugs are linked to failing health and possible side effects which could ultimately cause more damage than good. We all have seen those infamous commercials outlining the terrible side effects while actors portray a happy harmonious lifestyle. The commercials are very misleading as the side effects are expeditiously read while the patient appears to be enjoying the benefits of a certain drug. Well for some their life can be enhanced by these drugs because their health is in such dire straits. But we all want to steer as clear from those prescription drugs as possible in our lifetime. Using culinary herbs and spices in the kitchen is a great way to make your food tasty while boosting immunity and activating anti-inflammatory agents to increase the movement of waste out of your system and heal the body internally.

Below you will find some herbs and spices that are easy to incorporate into your next meal. Bon Appetite!

- **Ginger Root:** Ginger is a superfood high in antioxidants, used as an anti-sickness remedy for hundreds of years as it contains volatile oils, such as gingerol, that are known to stimulate saliva and gastric functions in our digestive system. Add ginger to hot water to assist with relieving symptoms of a cold and it aids in indigestion as well. Ginger has been known as a belly fat buster to melt stubborn visceral fat around the stomach.

- **Turmeric Herb:** One of my all-time favorites. Turmeric is arguably the most powerful herb found on the planet. It contains a healing compound called curcumin. It has been suggested to reverse damaged cells and specific diseases. A natural herb more powerful and healing than synthetic steroids, diabetes medication, chemotherapy, antidepressants cholesterol drugs, pain killers and so much more. Turmeric is also known to naturally whiten teeth and improve gum health. Add a little dash of turmeric to your life for overall health benefits.

- **Cinnamon**: Cinnamon is a more well-known spice, it's a spice we all have grown up with and more common to have in the kitchen cabinet, I am sure you have a bottle right now that you can go add a sprinkle to your next meal. Try adding a little to your warm, cold cereals, yogurt and a great addition to even a slice of peanut butter toast or your favorite shake. Cinnamon works directly on muscle cells to force sugar from the bloodstream which can be very helpful in treating Type 2 Diabetes. It also raises the good cholesterol (HDL). HDL helps remove the bad cholesterol from the body. Cinnamon has also been known to treat symptoms of Alzheimer's and Parkinson disease, these two maladies are neurological conditions that unfortunately at this present time are incurable. Treating these two conditions consist of symptom management which cinnamon helps to improve neurons and motor functions in these patients.

- **Cayenne spice:** Very good for firing up and boosting the metabolism. Also known for healing stomach tissue and stimulates the stomach's enzymes and helps to prevent stomach ulcers. Lowers bad cholesterol (LDL). An effective anti-inflammatory and pain remedy for everything from headaches to arthritis and sore muscles, as well as clearing nasal congestion while boosting immunity.

- **Oregano:** This herb is used to treat a wide range of conditions. Contains potent anti-bacterial, anti-fungal and anti-viral properties. Contains rosmarinic acid (also found in Rosemary spice). Kills parasites and stubborn fungal infections. Oregano is very high on the ORAC scale of antioxidants.

- **Black Pepper:** Loosens and unclogs pores, removes excessive sebum and impurities. Also contains antibacterial and antioxidant properties which help in removing acne and blackheads. Another benefit is black pepper lightens dark spots and aids in blood circulation of the skin to keep your skin looking refreshed.

  TRY IT: Black pepper and plain yogurt facial, allow the mask to dry and rinse off. Benefits: Tightens pores and evens the complexion.
  *Disclaimer: Test small section of skin to prevent skin irritation.

- **Cilantro/Coriander:** This power packed anti-inflammatory spice can reduce blood sugar and cholesterol and help digest fats. It's used to manage diabetes and lessen anxiety symptoms making it an all-in-one. Add the seeds to season meat, lentil and grain dishes, and the leaves are a convenient and great way to kick your salad or guacamole dip up 10 notches of yum.

- **Lavender Tea:** Most people think of lavender as being an essential oil for external use in baths and massages or aroma therapy only. However, the beautiful lavender flower buds can be dried and ingested in the form of tea. Used to treat mood and sleep disorders and helps with anxiety and depression along with soothing the nervous system. Eat lavender feel the purple power.

- **Fennel Seeds:** Fennel is one of the few plants that packs it all in. It is a vegetable, herb and spice. Fennel seeds have a distinct taste like licorice as they share the same volatile oil anethole. Teeming with dozens of phytochemicals including phytoestrogens that are found in estrogen like compounds found in plants. These properties help women to offset symptoms of monthly menstruation. The extract of fennel is labeled a nonsteroidal anti-inflammatory drug (NSAID) similar to ibuprofen but natural. In addition it may also help prevent and treat Alzheimer's, arthritis, cancer, colitis (inflammatory bowel disease), dementia, glaucoma, heart disease, high blood pressure, stroke and hirsutism (unwanted hair growth in women). Add fennel seeds to fruit salads. Dry and crush toasted fennel seeds and steep them in hot water to make tea. Fennel seeds complement many food ingredients taken from the Mediterranean diet (tomatoes, olives, olive oil, basil, lamb, and seafood). Try adding to scrambled eggs for great taste. Make a super powerful antioxidant salad dressing of spiced olives by marinating 2 cups olives in ½ cup extra-virgin olive oil and 1 teaspoon of fennel and oregano seeds and dried thyme over salad to boost your superfood power to the nth degree.

Chapter 16

Beau"TEA" In A Cup

Teatox To a Younger You......

Incorporate tea at least twice a day to literally soothe
and heal your mind body and soul. Teas are one of the
easiest ways to drink your way to longevity and health
they also offer a calming and relaxing start and or finish
to your day. Try some of the most powerful teas that
bind the hands of time and heal and preserve your beauty
inside out:

- **Matcha Green Tea** - If there was ever a magic
  potion that existed, Matcha green tea could
  certainly be the genie in the bottle. 1 cup of
  Matcha green tea is = to 10 cups of regularly
  brewed green tea in terms of antioxidants and
  nutritional content. There is so much to say
  about Matcha's awesome superfood powers, it is
  a very finely powered green tea mixed into liquid
  with powerful disease fighting properties. It

reduces the risk of cancer, boost metabolism, burns calories, reduces diabetes and Alzheimer's and improves liver functions.

- **Green Tea -** Since green tea is made from unfermented tea leaves, it is crowned the antioxidant jewel, extremely high concentration of polyphenol antioxidants which fight free radicals, damaged DNA, damage caused by aging, cancer, stroke and heart disease.

- **Rooibos Red Tea -** This comforting, low caffeine, this tea is one of my very favorite teas on earth. I absolutely love it! Red Rooibos tea is high in antioxidants aspalathin and nothofagin (phenolic antioxidants) which supports and improves cardiovascular health. This red tea inhibits angiotensin - converting enzymes to (ACE), ACE inhibitors help to relax blood vessels they prevent an enzyme in the body from producing a substance that narrows blood vessels and releases hormones that can raise your blood pressure. Red Rooibos tea also improves cardiovascular health.

- **Oolong Tea** - If you want healthier teeth and bones, sip Oolong tea. Beneficial in the prevention of tooth decay and the prevention of tartar build up on tooth enamel. This is why many Japanese dentists recommend slurping oolong tea for teeth and gum health. In addition, oolong has been linked to decreased bone deterioration, particularly osteoporosis in women.

- **Black Tea** - Black tea's process requires the leaves to be fermented in a highly humid environment which turns the leaves black which gives it a strong flavor. Packed with polyphenols that help in preventing the formation of potential carcinogens, antioxidants and flavonoids to prevent the oxidation of LDL cholesterol (good cholesterol), beneficial levels of caffeine promotes blood flow to the brain without over stimulating the heart, contains amino acid L-theanine that provides mental focus and clarity and helps to relax and prevent the negative stress hormone known as cortisol. Also has been known to treat depression.

- **White Tea** - White tea is the least processed of all the teas which yield the highest concentration of antioxidants and vitamins. It is touted as the "BEAU-TEA" tea in the eastern world. Lowers the risk for developing high blood pressure, extremely potent concentration of antioxidants, and reduces premature aging.

- **Ginseng Tea** - Ginseng is an all-around herb and tea known for its energy boosting properties, supports cognitive functions by increasing blood circulation, reduces cancer related fatigue, improves your sense of well-being, treats insomnia and stimulates the immune system.

Chapter 17

Super Herbs That Heal

Signed, Holistically, Healthy and Herbally Yours.........

Super herbs have long been used for their medicinal properties some herbs have the ability to slow aging or at least reduce some of the effects of aging. There are herbs that can boost energy, make the skin look younger, hair healthier and fuller and even improve memory. These are all important benefits for those of us over the age of 40 and beyond.

Not only can herbs make you look younger, they can also make you feel amazing. The ultimate goal is to feel alive, feel energized and look as great as you feel right? What good is it to look great and young but unable to keep up with the demands of your lifestyle? Try some of the following herbs to help supplement your well balanced diet:

Ginseng

Korean or American ginseng is very beneficial in preserving our youth and energy. This herb can reduce inflammation, increase mental and physical energy, reduce the effects of stress, enhance skin tone, and strengthen your immune system.

Gotu Kola

A native to India, Gotu Kola helps restore the skin and heal scars and blemishes. Gotu Kola is hailed as a memory herb, treats depression and lessens anxiety symptoms.

Jiaogulan (referred to as Southern Ginseng)

An herb widely used in China, Jiaogulan (Gynostemma) increases the production of the antioxidant superoxide dismutase. This keeps the body and skin looking young. It is a very powerful adaptogen, slows down aging and improves overall quality of life. It reduces bad cholesterol levels. In China this herb is also known as the herb of longevity.

Ashwagandha (Indian Ginseng)

Ashwagandha is very beneficial in treating hypothyroid symptoms. It promotes energy production, decreases fatigue, treats degenerative disorders, provides stress relief and manages the symptoms of arthritis.

St. John's Wort

This herb relieves depression and anxiety can also help to repair and heal the skin yielding a younger appearance. St. John's Wort is good for insomnia it aids in a good quality night's sleep which in turns improves your overall health on all levels.

Reishi Mushroom

A native to China and Japan, Reishi is said to promote long life and happiness. A very powerful adaptogen lowers stress, beneficial in reducing tumors from cancer, helps treat insomnia, boost the body's immune system against viruses. Lowers blood pressure and helps treat kidney, liver disease and cancer.

Red Clover

Red clover exhibits estrogen like effects in the body and can help to keep wrinkles away while assisting in keeping the skin beautiful and smooth.

Shilajit

Found in the Himalayan Mountains, Shilajit is a type of mineral paste found in cracks on the face of rocks that restores the body's health. It improves libido and the immune system. It also improves cognitive issues such as improving mental clarity, focus and concentration. Shilajit is a very powerful adaptogen that helps the body favorably deal and balance out internal stress.

Schizandra

The berries of the Schizandra are medically used as adaptogens to reduce stress. They boost the body's immune system to increase the resistance to disease. The berries also help to strengthen and normalize blood sugar and blood pressure. Excellent antioxidant in preventing premature aging. Treats physical exhaustion, promotes energy and a sense of well-being. Used externally, the berries help the skin retain moisture resulting in softer, smoother skin.

Bacopa Monnieri

Bacopa monnieri is a creeping marsh plant that is traditionally used as a nootropic (cognitive enhancer), for longevity, and to help with anxiety and depression. It's possible that the improved cognition is likely a result of the reduced anxiety. Bacopa is an effective adaptogen and can help you cope with stressful situations and decrease stress in all regions of the brain

Chapter 18

Eat Your ABC's

Open Up Wide......Say AHHHHHHHHH.......

As children we are taught our ABC's as a prerequisite for the foundation of learning and communicating with the world around us. It is ironic those same letters from our ABC's are also important vitamins we need in the foundation for our health and wellness throughout life.

Aging takes its toll on the vitamins our bodies produce and store over our life span. Each decade we are more prone to become deficient in critical vitamins and minerals needed to thrive and maintain our optimal levels of health. Multivitamins may not be the end all be all panacea to providing our bodies with all the necessary nutrients we need just as eating healthy foods alone cannot provide all of our nutritional needs. However, when a healthy balanced diet is supported with healthy quality supplements it works in tandem for optimal results.

A multivitamin is a great way to support a healthy well balanced diet. Eating a well-balanced diet can be a challenge on a daily basis. Vitamins that address specific and appropriate needs are required to supplement factors such as aging and a wide array of conditions. For instance, a pregnant and or lactating woman's body requires additional folic acid, a woman who is 40 and up will require more calcium and vitamin D3, a premenopausal and perimenopause woman will require various hormonal supplements as needed. As our bodies evolve and change with age we all need the appropriate nutrition that supports where we are currently in our lives and the aging process.

The body will show signs of normal wear and tear that's just a part of the journey of life. Our bodies are designed to age as it is a reality of life. However, there are certain areas on our bodies that age faster due to the delicate nature of the skin in these high risk areas. The skin around our eyes, neck, face and hands, lips and inner arms are thinner than other parts of our body. Those delicate areas are exposed to the harsh elements of the environment and age quicker. There is nothing like our skin telling our age before we can even introduce ourselves.

The vitamins below are extremely helpful in addressing common problems with aging skin:

1) **Vitamin E:** Fat-soluble compound that repairs dry and cracked skin when used as a lotion. When taken orally it helps the skin retain moisture and aids in healing wounds when applied directly to skin or by mouth. Vitamin E is an antioxidant that protects our body from the effects of free radicals. Free radicals seek out electrons from other cells, oxidizing them which results in damage in the cell and cell tissues as mentioned early. Vitamin E thins blood and prevents blood clotting (***warning*** do not take Vitamin E 2 weeks before surgery!!). Vitamin E also improves our immune system and assists with preservation of our genes. Good sources of vitamin E can be found in nuts, seeds, green leafy vegetables, and natural vegetable oils.

2) **Vitamin C:** Our skin is our largest organ of the entire body. Because it is our external organ it is underestimated in how critical our skin functionality is to life itself. Skin acts to waterproof, insulate, shield, guard and protect our body against extreme temperature, damaging sunlight, and harmful chemicals, as well as exudes antibacterial substances that prevent infection. Because our skin is an external organ it easily reveals the aging process. The appearance and outer shell of our skin largely depends on shape and firmness provided by collagen. Vitamin C intake improves the firmness and production of collagen, giving our skin a more firm and youthful appearance. The connective tissue is also important for wound healing. Fruits and veggies (especially citrus fruits and potatoes) are good sources of vitamin C. Additional good sources of vitamin C are found in: (sweet red/green peppers, swiss chard, turnip greens, spinach, broccoli, kiwi, strawberries, tomatoes and peas).

3) **Vitamin K:** Those dark circles around the eyes that literally show up overnight coupled with under eye bags can cause you to look tired and years older. Good grief is there any part of our body that does not scream or even whisper our age? The truth is every part of our body down to our eye balls reflects our current state of health. Dark circles and saggy skin under the eyes can be a result of leaking capillaries. Age is not the only factor that affects the appearance of the skin under and around the eyes. There are other factors such as heredity, hormones, allergies and other underlying health issues can be the culprit of darkening, puffy and wrinkled skin around the eyes. If you have dark circles due to pooling and clotting of blood, consume vitamin K or apply externally. Vitamin K aids in the constriction of capillaries to break up the tiny blood clots that form the dark circles. Our bodies produces very small amounts of vitamin K on its own but we are able to reap the benefits of vitamin K via the following foods: (kale, lettuce, spinach, and

broccoli, plums, dried prunes, grapes, rhubarb, avocados, kiwi and pears).

4) **Vitamin D:** If ever there were a vitamin that is underrated and often so often over looked is that good ole 4th letter in the alphabet vitamin D. One of the most important vitamins which our bodies needs in the fight against premature aging. As we age our bodies become less efficient in making vitamin D. Due to the fact vitamin D is fat soluble, the higher your body fat percentage the lower bioavailability in the body. In fact, obese individuals have 50% less bioavailability than non-obese individuals. Vitamin D deficiency has been linked to telomere shortening. Telomeres are plastic tips at the end of our chromosomes that protect our replicated DNA sequence pattern. Imagine the plastic caps at the end of a shoestring lace. Once that plastic tip on our shoestring lace gets tattered or comes off, it is a matter of time before the shoe string starts to fray and shred. Same analogy with the telomeres in our bodies. Telomeres fray leaving our cells exposed to

damage and aging. When telomeres undergo a permanent arrest it is called **senescence**. A few cells have a special enzyme called telomerase. Telomerase activates the rebuilding of cells. The lengths of our telomeres are used as a biological marker of age. It is believed the younger we are the longer our telomere length.

Below are factors that shorten and/or lengthen our telomeres:

- **Factors that shorten telomere length:**
  The following factors speeds up the aging process: Chronic stress, alcohol, smoking, lack of sleep, inflammation in the body, obesity and oxidative stress.

- **Factors that extend telomere length:**
  The following factors slow down the aging process: Vitamin D sufficiency, Omega-3 sufficiency, folic acid sufficiency, meditation and exercise. In a nutshell vitamin D helps promote the length and health of our telomeres. Be sure to get your required dosage of vitamin D.

Getting a little sunlight helps promote your body to make vitamin D. Due to the fact many may not get their required levels of healthy sun during winter months and individuals with darker skin (melanin actually slows the absorption of Vitamin D3) it is recommended you supplement with Vitamin D3 accordingly.

5) **Vitamin A:** One of the best anti-aging vitamins goes to the first letter in the alphabet. Vitamin A helps with aging in many ways to include preventing damage caused by free radicals. Internal oxidation of our cells caused by free radicals is believed to be a primary accelerator for age related degeneration. Topical solutions with Vitamin A (retinol) help to minimize fine lines and exfoliate dead skin cells to reveal younger tighter skin. The following foods are high in Vitamin A: (sweet potatoes, carrots, butternut squash, romaine lettuce, dark leafy greens such as kale, dried apricots, mango, cantaloupe, sweet red peppers and tuna).

6) **Vitamin B12:** Offers many anti-aging properties. Vitamin B-12 is one of the many essential nutrients that keep you feeling sharp, energetic and youthful. It is a very important factor in regulating the production of red blood cells, lack of B12 can often make you feel exhausted and fatigued. If you are experiencing lack of energy coupled with brain fog it is a possible telltale sign you could be lacking sufficient levels of vitamin B12 that promote oxygen in your cells. Vitamin B12 also plays a big role in the nervous system, think of it as Teflon or a protective covering for our nerve cells. If you are vitamin B12 deficient, your myelin coating slowly diminishes, leaving your nerve cells open and vulnerable to harm and communication breakdown. If you are found to have a vitamin B12 deficiency there are many ways to normalize your B12 levels from over the counter natural treatment or doctor prescribed vitamin B12 shots.

Chapter 19

Happy Healthy Hormones

Wake up your Thyroid..... Your Thyroid is not Connected to Your Thy bone..... (Laughs out Loud)......

I once asked a lady if she checked her thyroid. When she reached for her thigh and replied "Well my "thighs" have always been my problem area". I burst into laughter as her face revealed a perplexed look. I explained to her where here thyroid gland was located and informed her that the thyroid was not located in her leg and could very easily be an underlying factor in not seeing her desired weight loss results. Ok we both had a laugh on the thyroid's location in the body. However, the thyroid gland is NO laughing matter for so many who have thyroid issues. I recommended everyone get their thyroid levels checked.

Happily ever after hormones may be as elusive as a happily ever after marriage. In an ideal fairy tale world "Happily Ever After" exist. You are likely to find

Happily Ever After some place where a unicorn jumps over the rainbow in a pot filled with lucky charms, a rabbit's foot, four leaf clovers, a wish bone and a piece of chocolate. As we age our hormones need to be balanced and working harmoniously to keep our bodies functioning "Happily Ever After".

In the grand scheme of life, keeping fit and healthy relies on several factors and our hormones are often over looked. Many people try diet plan after diet plan of the "GET SKINNY NOW" claims they also believe if they exercise insanely that they can reach their health and fitness goals faster. The burnout is too real and you could never exercise insanely for a lifetime. Over exercising makes you susceptible to injury and exhaustion that weakens your immune system. The prime objective is to train to preserve your health not degrade it by over training and "Yo Yo" dieting which causes the body to be in a constant state of fluctuation that cause deviations in desired results and more harm than good. The truth is many people may not see their desired results due to unknown conditions stemming from their hormones and other possible genetic issues. It is true that our mind controls all of our body's functions. However, our hormones are next in rank and file acting as our body's inner thermostat controlling everything from our growth, metabolism, pregnancy cravings and lactation, reproductive organs, oxygen levels, glucose levels, sleep, PMS, fight or flight sensor, heart and blood pressure, and weight. It is recommended you see your doctor to do an overall health assessment to check your hormone levels.

Foods that Naturally Support Hormone Production

For LOW estrogen levels try eating some of the following foods:

Dried fruits: Dried apricots, dates and prunes, can help balance estrogen levels. These fruits contain phytoestrogens which mimics the way estrogen is used in the body. Note the drying process concentrates all the fruit to include the sugar so although you will get more vitamins and nutrients the natural sugar content is higher versus eating just fresh fruit that has not been dried.

Flaxseeds: Flaxseeds are a very effective way to increase your estrogen levels naturally. It is good to note flaxseed's omega-3's are not the same omega-3's from animal sources such as salmon. A very convenient and easy way to consume flaxseeds is in liquid or seed form.

Thyroid Deficiency and/or Excessive Thyroid Production

If there ever was the big "T" that applies to our hormones it certainly would stand for the thyroid. The thyroid gland is a part of our endocrine system and controls many body functions. It makes and stores hormones that help regulate everything from heart rate, blood pressure, body temperature to the rate at which our food we consumed is converted into energy known as our metabolism. The thyroid is essential for every cell in our body. The thyroid uses Iodine, mineral found in some food and iodized salt, to make its hormones. The two most important hormones the thyroid creates are thyroxine (T4) and triiodothyronine (T3). The pituitary gland produces (TSH) which stimulates hormone production by the thyroid gland. In addition, the thyroid gland also makes the hormone calcitonin which is involved in calcium metabolism and stimulating bone cells to add calcium to our bones.

The 3 Major Forms of Thyroid Conditions Are:
1. Hyperthyroidism
2. Hypothyroidism
3. Thyroiditis

Hyperthyroidism - Overactive thyroid production:

Symptoms include: Sudden weight loss, enlarged thyroid gland, menstrual issues, fatigue and muscle weakness, tremors, sweating, hair loss and increased appetite.

Foods to Consume with Hyperthyroidism

Berries - (strawberries, blueberries, raspberries and blackberries).
Berries are packed with antioxidants to keep your immune system strong.

Broccoli - This green vegetable is a part of the goitrogen family - these are foods that can decrease the amount of thyroid hormone your thyroid produces.

Yogurt: Hyperthyroidism that has been untreated can eventually lead to bone loss which can weaken your bones and run the risk of developing osteoporosis. You can potentially prevent this by eating 3 servings of yogurt per day or other dairy foods of your choice.

Turkey: Weight loss is common to hyperthyroidism. Ensuring you are eating enough protein will assist with maintaining a healthy weight with hyperthyroidism. Turkey is a good source of lean protein to help with weight maintenance. In the event you do not eat meat, you can opt for alternatives such as beans, lentils, veggies, tofu, nuts and tempeh (which pack approximately 30 grams of protein). Other alternatives are premium quality plant based protein shakes.

Avoid: Refined flour (found in bread, desserts, pizza and pasta), refined sugars (baked goods, cereal, sweet drinks, and dairy products) and fast food sources.

Hypothyroidism – Underactive Thyroid Production

Symptoms include: extreme fatigue, constipation, dry skin, brittle nails, thinning hair, irregular menstrual cycles, intolerance to cold temperatures and depression and memory problems. A common diagnosed thyroid disease is Hashimoto's an autoimmune disorder where the thyroid does not make the proper amount of thyroid hormones and eventually runs out if not managed appropriately.

Typically when you are diagnosed with Hashimoto's, synthetic steroids are prescribed (Synthroid) to assist in the thyroid's production. Unfortunately, like many prescription drugs the side effects are not desirable and often times introduce new health issues as a result of steroids. There are alternative natural treatments to hypothyroid disorders managed via naturopathy. Please consult with a holistic naturopathic doctor for more alternative treatment options.

Foods to Consume with Hypothyroidism

Salmon

Unmanaged hypothyroidism can increase the risk for heart disease as a result of higher levels of low-density lipoprotein (LDL), the "BAD" cholesterol. "Omega-

3's are known to decrease inflammation, helps with lowering the risk for heart disease.

Nuts

Nuts are a very good source of selenium in particular macadamia, brazil and hazel nuts offer a powerful punch of selenium. Selenium promotes proper functioning of the thyroid. Because nuts are very high in fats, be sure not to over indulge a handful will do the job just fine.

Fresh Fruits and Vegetables

An early symptom of hypothyroidism is weight gain. Low-calorie, high-density foods such as fresh produce are the cornerstone of every successful weight loss program especially with hypothyroid. Include fresh fruits and veggies with each meal if possible (supplement when needed). Specific foods such as blueberries, cherries, sweet potatoes, and green peppers are very rich in antioxidants, these foods are known to lower the risk of heart disease.

***Note: Hypothyroid leads to diminished levels of iodine therefore, broccoli and cabbage should be limited to 5 ounces/day because they can block the thyroid's ability to absorb iodine.

PMS - Premenstrual Syndrome

From time to time women may experience various symptoms from our monthly cycles that get a bad rap. If we are easily annoyed and irritated and our emotions seem to be out of sync it is usually during a certain time of the month as our hormones are preparing our bodies for a possible pregnancy. This process throws our body into a state or raging hormones where we may experience everything from mood swings, bloating, headaches, constipation, food cravings, tenderness in breast, to cramps. If you are fortunate to conceive a adorable bundle of joy (baby) you can appreciate your 9 months where your cycle is disrupted to support your pregnancy. Oh but you are certainly not out of the waters as pregnancy hormones are just as brutal. However, every month many of us are not looking to conceive that bundle of joy and our bodies gives us a small little consolation prize sometimes known as PMS (humor at its best). Stop!!!! Before you go grab that bag of salty chips loaded with sodium or that indulgent slice of decadent chocolate cake below are some healthier options to help ease symptoms of PMS:

Brussels Sprouts, and Artichokes

Adds fiber and helps with constipation, gas and bloating due to the high water content in these foods. These vegetables also reduce water weight.

Wheat Berry, Quinoa and guess what???? Popcorn (Yeap)

Complex carbohydrates boost serotonin (the feel good hormone) in addition to providing a boost of energy. Many times our menstrual cycle impacts our sleep habits. Did you know without the proper amount of sleep your body is more prone to pain and the smallest disturbances at night as well as weight gain? So if you suffer from cramps the pain will seem a lot more intense as you lay wide awake counting the number of sheep at night. Eating banana's help to regulate our body's natural rhythm so have a couple of bananas throughout the day to rest a little easier at night.

Pumpkin Seeds/Pumpkin Spice

Pumpkin seeds/spices are one in a long list of ingredients that are underrated and underappreciated. We normally have a taste during the fall for one of pumpkins tasty treats, either a pumpkin pie or maybe a pumpkin latte. The seeds of pumpkins are full of magnesium. Magnesium is believed to relax blood vessels which alleviate headaches. Try baking some pumpkin seeds and sprinkling over a salad, baked kale or grab a handful and enjoy. Pumpkin spice can be added to protein shakes for an added zing.

Fibroids and Hormones

It is believed that hormones play a big role in the development of uterine fibroids. Doctors believe there may be a genetic link to fibroids. A primary focus is the connection between estrogen, xenoestrogens (chemically similar to estrogen but found in growth hormones in foods), progesterone and cortisol. Chronic stress and elevated levels of cortisol in the body have also been linked to fibroids in women. The following are natural food sources to help prevent and manage fibroids:

Unprocessed Grains

White foods such as starchy breads, pasta, and rice increase the production of insulin in the body which influences the way estrogen is metabolized. This may increase the risk for fibroids. To improve your uterine health and possibly protect you from developing fibroids "THINK THE COLOR BROWN!" Eat nutritious brown oats, brown rice, wild rice, quinoa and barley. It is also worthy to note, although a healthy diet cannot cure or prevent hyperthyroidism due to genetic implications. Eating the aforementioned foods may help manage and ease hyperthyroidism symptoms.

Disclaimer: Consult your doctor if you have a history of thyroid disorders in your family or you suspect you may be suffering from symptoms of: (Hypothyroidism/Hyperthyroidism). A licensed nutritionist/dietician is highly recommended to provide nutritional meal plans the suggestions below are not to substitute or override professional expert knowledge and medical advice.

Chapter 20

Movement the Dance of Life

Don't Let the Daisy's Grow Under Your Toes.......
Movement is Life's Dance Partner and the Universe is the Music
that Choreographs our SOULS ....

"KEEP IT MOVING" is more than just a trite
expression it is the key metaphorically as well as literally
to move through, move past, and move on through life's
inevitable ups and downs. This applies to both our
mental and physical ability to keep moving. When we
keep our mind sharp and stay active enough to burn
those calories it keeps our bodies young healthy. It is
thought that once the mind and body become too idle we
waste our life moments and loose minutes off our
lifespan. I am not sure if you can even quantify something
of this nature but you sure can directly correlate health
and wellness to the mind and body being physically fit
enough to live a quality lifestyle. Sit too long and your
aching by the time you get up.....sleep too long by the
time you wake up you're feeling even more fatigued

....allow your mind to run idle and when the time comes to focus you can't concentrate enough to be productive (raised hand been there more times than I like to admit).

The body needs to be active during the day to promote healthy blood circulation to all of our vital organs. Sitting, laying and or standing still too long restricts our blood flow. We all have experienced those nagging sensations of prickly pins and needles and sometimes numbness in our extremities. We always hear someone complain about their arm or leg falling asleep. Your mother warned you not to sit legs crossed because it stops the blood from circulating. Most times those pins and needles can be associated with improper sitting. In more serious cases pins and needles (paresthesia) can be attributed to some other underlying health issue and should be checked by your healthcare provider.

Start looking for opportunities to become more active. Moving can be anything from getting up to stretch periodically, taking the stairs or parking the car and taking the road less traveled. It does not have to be any complicated workout routine, you don't even have to drive to the gym or even leave your home but, you need to be as active as possible every day for the rest of your life. SO GET UP! GET OUT! AND KEEP IT MOVING!

Chapter 21

The Gift of Exercise

Exercise is our bonus chromosome to combat aging.....
The "E-FACTOR".....Exercise is Nature's Natural Medicine
for the Mind, Body and Soul....

Can you move without exercising? The fact of the matter is you can move without it being considered exercise. Moving unconsciously is considered a physical activity and qualifies as being active. We all need to be as active as we can as we go throughout our day. Any movement can technically be considered exercise but when done intentionally for a dedicated duration of time your body reaps the full benefits. There are benefits to conscious deliberate exercise. You are willfully using your mind to complete a physical activity. The mind is sending messages to every part of your body to work harder. Never underestimate the conscious aspect of exercising. Of course it is good to be active everyday however, when you decide to move with purpose and intent it requires a mind, body, soul connection which trains your brain. Deliberate exercising trains your mind when your body is telling you "We don't need to work out today". When you make the decision to exercise you are exercising full control of the strongest muscle in your body. The mind is required to be consistent to make your diet and exercise habit forming. Daily activity helps support an active lifestyle however deliberate exercising will improve every aspect of your life. You will start to feel more confident. Your mind and body is constantly duking it out in a power struggle. When the mind is exercised the body aligns. It is not the other way around. You do not exercise to change your mind. You may think your body is telling your mind we don't feel like exercising but in all actuality your mind has the overall originating prevailing thoughts of not wanting to exercise. When you systematically work on your mind the body is submissive to every thought. Your successes and your failures are an end product and a result of your current mindset.

Movement allows the body to burn calories and is essential in aiding our metabolism. Ok I don't want you to stress out or get caught up with whether or not you are exercising properly. The great thing about getting up and moving is every step and physical activity counts. It is a step in the right direction. There is not some exercise holy grail you need to follow. Remove any doubts and negative feelings surrounding moving your body. Everybody will not be the gym rat. Everybody will not run a 26.2 marathon. Everybody will not jump on the latest exercise challenge. You absolutely do not need to step foot in a gym to work out and exercise. Sometimes improving our health can take place in as little as one foot in front of the other. Exercising at home can provide for quick easy no fuss workouts. No need to get in the car and drive to a gym your home is a great place to move and work up a good sweat. Get up off that couch ....out of your favorite cozy chair....out of the bed. Make a space in your home to workout. Do not put anything in this space (with the exception of exercise equipment), make it sacred a place you go to move and exercise at any time. When you set aside the space make sure you only use it to work out.

Do not add the extra temptation of bailing out of your workout because you have to move furniture and clean up your work out area. It becomes easy simple and a habitual habit when your area is READY, SET and GO!

Cleaning the house to your favorite song can serve as just as much exercise as a gym workout. Before you know it you're moving and dancing all around the house, reaching, bending, pulling, wiping, sweeping, mopping, sweating and working off those calories....and my favorite added benefit is your house is nice and clean when you are done.

Exercise is one of the most effective and efficient ways to stay healthy and young. Diet and exercise together becomes the key to unlock your door to vitality and longevity. You are in full possession of your key. Nobody owns the key it is in your hands. Exercising not only keeps your joints in good working order, it maintains the skin's elasticity and sweating flushes out harmful toxins. So how many days does one have to exercise per week? I would personally recommend you do at least 20mins to 30 minutes of exercising daily for weight maintenance and from 45 minutes to 1 hour or longer if you are exercising to lose weight on a daily basis. Whether you are maintaining your weight or trying to lose weight, I suggest working out 4/5 times per week.

Exercising does not have to feel like a chore. It absolutely does not have to be punishment for not sticking to your meal plan. Pick something you enjoy doing and go for it. Cardio is needed more as we age to keep our heart beating healthy and strong. Strength, resistance and flexibility training should be incorporated to build that nice lean muscle tone which makes our bodies look healthy and fit.

People who exercise age slower and look younger than their counterparts who do not exercise simple as that. Exercising releases stress and our endorphins kick in which makes us feel happier and more energetic as we go through life. This fact alone should be more incentive to make exercising a daily lifestyle staple. There is a huge relationship between exercising and combating depression and mood enhancement.

The really awesome thing about exercising is you can start where you are NOW. Start slow small incremental steps take it one day at a time. Do not focus on how long it will take you to see your results. Focus on your daily wins. You win each and every day you make healthier choices over your life.

Chapter 22

Create a Youthful Loving Mindset

Plant Fruitful Seeds of Beautiful Thoughts and Reap the True Harvest of your Brain Food ......

How many times have you heard people or you may even be guilty yourself of saying: "I am getting OLD"? "I am too old to start", "I am too old to lose the weight", "I am too old to feel young again", "I am too old to start a new routine", "I am too old to change my eating habits" or "I am too old to inspire anyone else to change". If you say this to yourself over and over it will manifest 10 fold. You have sowed the seed of death essentially over your own health and ultimately your life. The patterns that show up in our lives are rehearsed over and over in our mind until they play out in our realities. The body aligns with what you think and speak and it will manifest negatively or positively on your health. So stop speaking death over your very existence. If there was one saying about aging that I would banish, it would be "40 is over the hill". What hill? Where is this hill? There is not a hill or a mountain that can't be moved when you change your thoughts. How many times have you heard this misconception? People who take care of their health do not subscribe to this defeatist attitude and mindset. Take control over your mind. Speak words of STRENGTH, INTEGRITY, RESOLVE, DETERMINATION AND LOVE. Create in you a new mindset for your new improved lifestyle.

So many people like to swap horror stories about reaching 40. They can't wait to tell you with enthusiasm how bad it gets when you hit your 40 year anniversary on this earth. The negative talk about weight gain, slower reflexes and mental decline are always at the top of the list. Very seldom do you hear people speak of having more energy and gusto for life beyond their 40's. It is as if they have settled and accepted what others say and not what they believe they could change. Yes I have heard it all, they say 40 is when gravity finally catches you and ties you down and makes you eat cupcakes (smile). Well I had more than a few of those cupcakes in my life, and I have yet to surrender my thoughts to 40 being over the hill or banishing cupcakes completely out of my life.

Our brain is a very powerful instrument it will cosign on every thought good, bad and/or indifferent. Fill your mind with ageless thoughts of health and wellness all around you.

Visualize yourself HAPPY, HEALTHY and last but not least WEALTHY! It is easy for people to want to be wealthy. There are people out there who think it is much easier to become a millionaire than to become healthy and fit. Health and Wealth are cut from the same cloth. Both consist of focusing your mind and positioning yourself through mindset, habits, dedication that leads to results. One outlines your business mindset and the other outlines your health blue print. Visualize yourself healthy and wealthy. Not one over the other. Implant those thoughts in your mind allow them to recur over and over. Let's refocus back specifically to having or acquiring an ageless spirit. Being young at heart and spirit is what really resonates with people. Sure maybe we have gotten to the point we can no longer keep up with the number of gray strands on our heads. Accept age as a virtue! One person's grey hair is another person's silver streak. I personally love the color silver. The view we hold and form of ourselves should be rooted in self-love, self-worth and self-appreciation. Once your outlook on life changes, you will start to move different in the world down new paths of renewed self-awareness, self-acceptance and self-discovery. Each year should teach us the beauty of every second of life. Reprogram your mind to see the good in aging and your brain will work in unison with you to keep your body, mind and spirit ageless. Feed your mind positive thoughts and affirmations. As a matter of fact, one of my favorite tea mugs declares; "I AM Aging To Perfection". Every time I take a sip I believe this with every fiber of my being. The saying goes "Age AINT NOTHING BUT A NUMBER". Age takes into consideration your mindset, healthy living, your strength, your thirst for knowledge, acceptance of self and your ability to see the beauty in life at any age.

Below are some very good affirmations you should make a habit of speaking daily. You may be thinking how do affirmations work or why are they so important? Are they some sort of esoteric, hocus pocus mumbo jumbo? Well if you are not too familiar with God's universal laws it is quite normal to question whether affirmations actually work. Our brain is constantly overwhelmed with so many images, social media post, unworthy news articles, other's beliefs and opinions we need a deliberate method to get the information that matters to our brain. Our brain has what is known as a Reticular Activating System (RAS), which is essentially our filter to allow the necessary information we need to form as well as support positive habits and thoughts. So it's real simple when we speak daily affirmations or focus on good thoughts it sends a clear concise signal or message alerting our brain that this affirmation is essential and what we desire over the inundated negative clutter. So it goes like this, you speak your affirmation(s) and your Reticular Activating System immediately kicks in to narrowly focus your attention on everything relating and supporting your affirmation(s) cementing these thoughts into your mental concrete.

Your RAS is much like your x ray vision your bull's eye so to speak that reveals new opportunities, resources, people, places and things and new thought processes to reach your declared goals. It is not rocket science. It is a methodology that is long standing with biblical context.

Speak these affirmations out loud and or record your voice repeating these affirmations and listen to the recording at night or in the morning anytime you need instant brain food for positive thought. This is your "To Do Task"!!!!!

- I Am Beautifully Created In God's Image
- I Am Young In Mind, Body and Soul
- I Love Everything About Myself
- I Am Full of Life and Enthusiasm To Live A long Healthy Life
- My Body Keeps me Strong and Healthy
- I Am the Only One That Can Take The Best Care of Myself
- I Believe That I Am Continuously Evolving Into The Best Version(s) of Me
- I Love Me
- I Am Love

- I Feel Alive and Amazing
- I Am Enough
- I Love Spending Time With Me
- I Am Worth It
- I Am Living a Life Full Of Abundance
- I Am Living a Healthy Life Of Longevity
- I Am Healthy, Wealthy and at Peace with Life

Chapter 23

Create a Vacation Life

How Are You? I Am Just Beachy!
A Little Vacation Mindset Does Not Always Require Travel, but
Certainly Goes a Long Way......

Our ability to learn how to master calmness throughout life's choppy waters, and proactively eliminate stressful situations in our lives may be easier said than done. Everyone loves a picture of a nice serene white sand beach, at the edge of beautiful blue azure waters. Clear skies, pretty flowing palm trees, and high back beach chair. We can even envision a yellow umbrella sticking out of a pineapple nicely adorning the rim of a frosty cold Pina colada with our name written all over it. We imagine the misty breezes off of the beach shores lightly sprinkling us as we lay honey baked to perfection. The sun hands us a little souvenir of rotisserie tan lines to take back home as a gentle reminder of our dream vacation. We envision ourselves lying on a colorful bright beach towel enjoying the sun's rays and crashing waves as we relax. Sometimes that is exactly what we need a vacation to get away. We all need some downtime from our busy lives from our routines where we fly on autopilot until we are sputtering about on exhaust fumes. We are frazzled, tattered and wish we had not used up all of our personal days so we could book the next plane to some fantasy island where rest, relaxation and rejuvenation awaits our soul. Vacations are certainly nice opportunities to enjoy some much needed R & R if you are fortunate to have the luxury of money and time off. Vacations never last long enough before we need to schedule yet another get away. As soon as the plane lands we are back to our reality our daily grind which is the very source as to why we need a vacation to begin with. Creating time to revive our soul and preserving our sanity and health in between those vacations are extremely important in maintaining a balanced lifestyle. Instead of waiting to cram your Zen into a week's worth of rest and relaxation, create daily rituals that replenish your well spring. The ability to tap into your Zen mode of reprieve from your daily rigors really helps replenish and balance our hectic lifestyles. Set aside some time for yourself just 'YOU". Grab a hold of that favorite novel you been meaning to pick back up. Schedule that much needed massage you deserve it. What is it that you love to do but can never find the time? Everybody seems to get a spot on your "TO DO" list except for the person who sits down to write the list that is "YOU". Anytime is a great time to revisit your interest that gets shoved, pushed, moved, tossed and left off of your "TO DO" list. Don't pencil yourself in. Make yourself a PRIORITY! Find the time, cut off all the notifications we get reminding us of their importance. The urgent voicemails, the high priority work related email alerts, the social media notifications, and all the smart phone reminders. Today more than ever we have so many distractions that have become accepted as our norm and status quo. Some people will even proclaim that we all need to become better at multitasking. At some time in our lives we need to do somethings simultaneously as life often has a way of throwing balls at us to see how well we are able to keep them in the air. Typically the balls that fall are the ones we really should be focusing our attention on. Life should not be about how well you can juggle your balls in the air for an extended period of time but how well you can consistently balance out your lifestyle on a daily basis. Life is better when we are focusing and concentrating on those things that are essential to our lives and our well-being. Drop the guilt trip of not being a good juggler or talented at multitasking. Multitasking is overrated!

There is no gold medal or first place because you can disorient your brain's neurons and synapses or retrain your brain to become unfocused. Yes I will go on record to say multitasking is practically stealing your brain's firing signals. When we multitask all day it literally changes the way our brains are wired to cement and archive information. Our ability to concentrate and focus on a thought is actually a form of exercise for our minds. We have two hands to hold and anything that does not fit snug and tight in our grasp should get placed in the non-essential folder. Listen, I am not speaking about the peaks and valleys in our lives where we may have some uncertain life changes or issues causing us to dive in head first, into responsibilities and task that require us to use both hands, arms and maybe even balancing something on our head.

Unfortunately or fortunately there will be times where we will have to dig deep and go all in. For instance, a death or maybe a new edition to the family, a big move to another city, or a new promotion or starting your own business these can be very stressful times where we need to employ all hands on deck, full court press for a specified timeframe. However, every day should not be code red high alert and reactive days you should task yourself with the gift of prioritization. Prioritize your most important commitments and take anything off your plate that are nonessential and metaphorically kindly eat them for leftovers the next day. Learn The Art of Saying NO! Learn The Art of Saying YES to Living a Well Balanced Inspired LIFESTYLE!

Chapter 24

Forgiveness Is Life's Youth Serum

Drink Forgiveness Serum to Revitalize Your Health and Life.......Cheers!!!

Many times we tend to hold onto things that have deeply hurt us. We may forgive to a certain degree but we never forget, otherwise how on earth would we remember who to hold grudges against. Unsurprisingly this is some people's train of thought when it comes to forgiveness. Are you keeping a long laundry list of people who have disappointed you, let you down or wronged you? Or are you holding your own feelings hostage to situations and circumstances that you have not forgiven yourself for? Those life experiences that caused us to be on guard, build a fortress around our heart is like drinking our own poison over and over. Forgiving others for how they treated us, betrayed our trust, spoke disparaging words or did not keep their promise will allow you to live free. Holding grudges and continuing to rehash the situation over and over creates a chain reaction in your mind similar to our fight or flight reflexes. Our natural inclination to fight or flight is our ability to perceive danger and react accordingly within secs. It is our built in security system. These sensors get stimulated even if there is no real imminent danger in sight. So when you are imagining the hurtful situation or harboring resentment in your heart each time it sets these alarms off in your mind. The brain alerts the amygdalae activating the bad stress hormones known as cortisol into our system. The nervous system becomes aware of these neurotransmitters setting off red flags to the sympathetic nervous system.

Your body is now in a high state of emergency and is focused on survival mode sending the body into a state of red alert. When the body is in survival mode the digestive system stops, saliva glands slow, blood pressure raises, pupils dilate, and your heart rate increases. If this state continues over and over it begins to cement aging within our cells. Keeping your mind, heart and soul free to forgive allows your body to stay in a harmonious state that helps prevents premature aging and many other unwanted health maladies.

Forgiveness Is a Choice!!!!!!!!!!!

Forgiveness is a choice we consciously make not to wallow in self-pity and not to stay in a perpetual state of fight or flight. Most times it is very hard to forgive and forget on our own. In order to really forgive and heal from hurtful situations we need help from our highest power (God). Don't try to forgive on your own strength or else you may never be able to forgive to completely transform your life through the power of forgiveness. Unleash your power of forgiveness. Forgiveness does not happen overnight it is a process. Do not worry yourself about your process of forgiveness as everybody will have a different path and timeline that provides closure to their own particular situation. Keep working towards forgiving so that you will be free to HEAL, LIVE and LOVE the LIFE you deserve.

Below are some steps to help you start your process of forgiveness and live your life free of resentment.

- Ask God to help you, let God know your honest feelings
- Allow yourself to process your feelings and emotions and Do Not try and rush the process

179

- Understand the importance of forgiveness for you and never think of it as gifting the other party their innocence
- Release the feeling of resentment towards the person especially if that person is you
- Comfort yourself with positive images surrounding the situation
- Write down the infraction and burn the paper and say Goodbye!

Chapter 25

Create a Life Full of Your Passions

Don't Just Follow Your Passion.....Live a Passion Filled Purposed Life!......

We have all come across passion filled people who have an enthusiasm for living . Maybe it's you who inspires others with your passion for living. Somebody may have felt inspired by the way you approach life or how you have triumphed from unfortunate circumstances in your life. Following your passion is not as important as living a life filled with love and purpose and things that bring your soul joy and peace of mind. People may not see what you give your time and resources to behind the scene or on the other hand they may have witnessed your soul glowing as you go about your life helping and being there to support people in their time(s) of need. When people do not cultivate their own self-interest and passion they lose a lot of their zeal and zest for life and it takes a toll on their well-being and permeates through their life's journey. Finding purpose in your life makes you happier and healthier and gives every day meaning to why God choose specifically you for your life journey. Having a sense of purpose will improve your productivity and positive outlook on life whereby making you feel more confident and self-assured.

People who kick about aimlessly without purpose are more prone to depression and living an unfulfilled life. Set goals for your life, goals allow us to keep learning, growing and feeling a sense of accomplishment. You should always be setting new goals. Write your goals down, make them happen!

The beautiful thing about aging is the fact you continue to get the opportunity to grow and learn in life which is its own reward. Each day gives us a free score card, it is up to you to score at your own dreams. The game is being played in real time that is right now. The only time that really matters on the clock is "THE NOW".

Planning and analyzing has its place and benefits but failure to act in "THE NOW" is primarily what stops people from seeing their dreams manifest into reality. Get up and tap into your purpose and drive and live a full life of passion filled moments. Don't just leave your footprints in the sand, stomp your footprints in the concrete to last forever.

Chapter 26

Skinspirational

Beauty May Be Only Skin Deep.....
But True Beauty is Being Confident in the Skin You're In......

Some of the first signs of aging show up on our skin.
Our skin is critically important and our largest organ that
covers our entire body and acts as everything from
protecting our internal organs to filtering out the toxins in
our body. It's our first line of defense against free
radicals scavenging our cells. A very quick easy way to
preserve our skin is to simply drink more water as well as
eat foods with a high percentage of water and oxygen
content. The body is comprised of water weight and
weight from our bones, muscles and organs. Hydration
is vital for our body to function properly and your body's
water ratio is an indication and measure of good health.

Of course wrinkles and dark circles and eye bags
(raccoon eyes) are a sure sign of how our body is aging.
Take two fingers and perform the pinch and pull test.

Pull your skin and notice how long it takes your skin to bounce back in place. If your skin immediately bounces back it shows your skin's elasticity is still healthy and strong. When you perform the pinch and pull test with the skin under our necks, around our eyes and skin inside our upper arms you will notice it takes longer to return to its normal state. This is partly due to this skin being thinner, thin skin matures at a faster rate and loses elasticity before other parts of our body.

Below are some good things to implement into your daily regimen to improve your overall health and improve the look and texture of your skin:

Alkaline water: Drink alkaline water. Drinking more water is a quick easy way to enhance your health on the spot. Alkaline water cleanses the body of acidity. When the body is in a normal alkaline state the cells function properly and keeps your skin's pH levels normal, revealing a more youthful complexion.

Sunscreen: Wearing sunscreen helps prevent those fine lines appearing much sooner than later. Dermatologist recommends wearing SPF 30+ for mature skin to protect and prevent damage and skin cancer. There is no such thing as being over protective with your skin it is ok to bump the SPF level up to 50.

Vitamin C: Vitamin C is one of the best anti-aging properties for mature skin to fight premature aging. Another name for vitamin C is ascorbic acid, it is a water soluble nutrient with tremendous antioxidant qualities that kicks starts and maintains your immune system and works to synthesize collagen levels. Vitamin C is the gem of all gems, it protects our bodies from oxidative damage. It's fine to maybe skip the apple for a few days and replace with an orange or a grapefruit. Squeeze a little lemon or lime in your water daily up the ante on your Vitamin C intake.

Astaxanthin: A very potent aquatic carotenoid that jumps to the front of the line of antioxidants. It is known for its anti-oxidative artillery, which improves everything from cardiovascular health, stabilizing blood sugar levels and fighting cancer. Astaxanthin is what gives salmon its deep pink color and also gives salmon the strength and endurance to swim up rivers and waterfalls for days. You can find astaxanthin in supplement form, it can be taken internally. This ingredient has been finding its way into sun screen lotions due to its potent ability to absorb ultraviolet rays. It also reduces damage to the body's DNA.

Collagen: The loss of collagen is a big factor in our skin's aging process. It is the glue to keeping the body nice, tight and firm. The Greek translation of collagen is in fact "glue". It is the predominant protein that builds the structure of our skin, tendons, joint cartilage, organs, and bones. Add some collagen supplements to your diet. (Note: For optimal absorption consume collagen with hydrolyzed types I and III).

Tips For Improving Skin Tone and Texture

Tip 1: Organic Coffee Bean Scrub

Try a nice invigorating organic unroasted coffee bean facial scrub also can be used on body to stimulate blood flow and improve the skin's elasticity. You can also purchase coffee beans in the form of oils. Coffee Arabica Seed Oil is extracted by cold pressing green coffee beans it has a very high concentration of essential fatty acids, sterols, and vitamin E makes it potent and helpful in fighting skin damage and photo aging it also has great inflammatory properties in the use of skin disorders.

Tip 2: Dry Brushing

The areas that we tend to neglect, are the areas that are covered up during the winter until the summer makes its debut. We spend a lot of attention and time on our face of course it is what everybody sees first. But the rest of our body tends to get overlooked and underappreciated. Dry brushing helps to exfoliate the skin's surface and it improves the appearance of the skin due to increased blood circulation. It also stimulates your lymphatic system and eliminates cellular waste. It helps to soften fatty deposits underneath the skin known as cellulite and keeps the skin plump.

Tip 3: Greek Yogurt, Raw Honey Matcha Green Tea Facial

Natural facial mask are an inexpensive way to improve the texture of your skin without paying the big bucks at a spa. Yogurt acts as an antibacterial that boost the natural bacteria on the skin. Honey is very beneficial in healing as well as hydrating the skin. Matcha green tea is very powerful and anti-oxidant rich and promotes skin rejuvenation and the skin's elasticity.

What you will need for this 3 ingredient natural mask:

1 teaspoon	Matcha Green Tea Powder
1 teaspoon	Raw Honey
1 teaspoon	Plain Greek Yogurt

Mix all the ingredients apply to face let dry for 10 minutes and rinse with cold water. Perform this facial 2-3 times per week

Chapter 27

Natural Raw Fermented Super Foods

Evoke your inner Popeye the Sailor Man... Toot Toot!!!! With Super Power Foods.....

We all witnessed Popeye the sailor man transform right before our eyes after he squeezed a can of his super food spinach that gave him 10 times the strength to defeat the big bully Bluto. Well there is a lot of truth to spinach being a super powerful food. In fact, the more natural and raw the food source, the more it acts as our very own Popeye within. These super foods fight on our behalf against the bullies that exact their toll on our cells, muscles and organs. Fresh organic vegetables are great but when they are fermented they become even more powerful and ultimately raise the bioavailability factor. When these same vegetables are converted by bacteria into super foods they become highly bioavailable meaning the rate at which our targeted organs, cells and systemic circulation absorb all the nutrients effectively.

Below are superfoods you need to get to the store and pick up at your earliest opportunity. Some listed will have to be ordered maybe via online or can be found in your local health food stores. However, there are plenty available at your neighborhood grocery store for purchase to immediately reap the benefits of your inner Popeye. A few of my favorites are:

Acai Berries: (Fruit) - Low in sugar, contains excellent amounts of iron, calcium, fiber and vitamin A.

Amaranth: (Grain) - Gluten free, the most nutritional of all the grains, very high in protein and minerals calcium, iron, phosphorous and carotenoids than most vegetables.

Beets: (Vegetable) - Good source of fiber, vitamin C, magnesium, and folate. Beets help to enrich the blood and blood circulation.

Black Garlic: (Vegetable) - Boost immunity, aids in digestive issues, anti-bacterial properties.

Bladderwrack: (Herb) - Stimulates thyroid gland, very high amounts of iodine, helpful with obesity and weight loss.

Buckwheat: (Grain) - Useful in managing high blood pressure, diabetes also lowers blood sugar levels and high in fiber.

Cactus Juice: (Fruit) - High in beta-carotene, vitamin B and C, iron, magnesium, rich in amino acids and taurine. Helps with weight loss, lowers LDL levels, high in antioxidants helps in preventing premature aging, soothes joint pain.

Chia Seeds: (Originates from plant) - Contains calcium, manganese and phosphorus and great source of essential omega-3 fats. Fights stubborn belly fat, improves heart health, helps maintain healthy bones and teeth.

Coconut Oil: (Considered fruit, nut and seed) - Very high in good fats medium-chained fatty acids (MCFA) contains caprylic acid, lauric acid and capric acid. Easy to digest and does not readily store in the body as fat.

Coconut is an instant energy booster and anti-microbial and anti-fungal.

Dark Chocolate: (Derived from the cocoa tree) 70% or higher - Very high in antioxidants, flavanols and vitamins. Lowers body mass, keeps your brain sharp, natural mood enhancer, improves eyesight, reduces inflammation, lowers blood pressure, fights sun damage and raises good cholesterol levels.

Hemp Seeds: (Originates from plant) - Hemp seeds are a great source of lean plant based protein and the highest of all the family of seeds packing a powerful punch of 10.3g of protein loaded with essential fatty acids of omega 3s and 9s, antioxidants. Hemp seeds promote weight loss, cardiovascular health, also high in magnesium, phosphorus, zinc and iron.

Kale: (Vegetable) - High in calcium, iron, beta-carotene, vitamin C and fiber. Lowers cholesterol levels, serves as a detox, rich with organic Sulphur compounds known to fight cancers (specifically colon cancer).

Flaxseeds: (Plant based) - High in omega-3 essential fatty acids great for heart health, lignans which have plant estrogen and antioxidants, fiber both insoluble and soluble. Flaxseed reduces the risk of certain cancers as well as cardiovascular disease.

Mangosteen Fruit: (Fruit) - Contains essential nutrients calcium, iron, magnesium, phosphorus, potassium, sodium, zinc, copper and manganese along with vitamin C, vitamin B12, vitamin A, thiamin, riboflavin, niacin, pantothenic acid, folate, folic acid, carotene and cryptoxanthin. All of these properties make mangosteen the queen of all fruits. The pericarp of mangosteen contains xanthones which are anti-cancer, anti-inflammatory and anti-bacterial. Mangosteen has been known to improve the following conditions: diabetes, menstrual issues, diarrhea, dysentery and is effective in weight loss.

Moringa Leaf: (Plant) - Moringa Leaf is very rich in phytonutrients, contains essential proteins, vitamins and minerals, rich in amino acids, also contains vitamins A, B1 (thiamine), B2(riboflavin), B3(niacin), B6, folate and ascorbic acid. Minerals include calcium, potassium, iron, magnesium, phosphorous, zinc and low in fat. Aids in everything from liver protection, diabetes, eye health, cardiovascular health, bone health, wound healing, sickle cell disease, anemia, obesity and building a strong immune system.

Olive Oil: (Drupe fruit) - One of the healthiest edible oils contains high concentrations of mono-unsaturated fatty acids to saturated fatty acids. Olive oil is beneficial in treating the following: depression, cholesterol, eliminating kidney stones, weight loss, preventing strokes, preventing Alzheimer's and Diabetes. Olive oil can also be used externally on the skin, hair, and nails.

Pink Himalayan Salt: (Rock salt) - A natural alternative to regular white table salt. Regular table salt goes through a process of bleaching and contains aluminum derivatives and other highly toxic ingredients. Pink Himalayan Salt is the purest salt on earth and contains over 84 minerals and trace elements, including calcium, magnesium, potassium, copper and iron. Benefits include: improving respiratory problems, balances the body's pH levels and contains iodine. Can be added to bath to promote detoxification, soothe soreness as well as used to purify the air, relieves sinuses, improves digestion, and reduces acid reflux.

Seaweed: (Green algae) - Very high in protein and minerals: iodine, calcium, iron, magnesium and more vitamin C than oranges, antioxidants, vitamins B and fiber, alpha linoleic acid and EPA, along with anti-viral, anti-bacterial. Seaweed has long been a powerful super food that potentially can reduce the risk of breast cancer and improve female fertility issues.

Spirulina: (Algae) - Contains one of the highest concentrations of chlorophyll of any food known. Known for its ability to break down toxins and heavy metals in the body and balance other trace minerals and help with gastrointestinal problems which makes it a great detox food. Helps diminish allergies and hay-fever, reduces blood pressure and cholesterol, helps controls symptoms of ulcerative colitis and packs a strong punch of antioxidants and anti-inflammatory characteristics.

Swiss Chard: (Vegetable) - Contains antioxidants, alpha and beta-carotene, lutein, zeaxanthin and choline. Swiss chard decreases the risk of many adverse health conditions such as obesity, diabetes and heart disease. It contains chlorophyll which has been shown to be effective at blocking cancer causing heterocyclic amines generated when foods are grilled at very high temperatures. It also contains the antioxidant alpha-lipoic acid which is known to lower glucose levels as well as beneficial in peripheral neuropathy.

Wheat Grass: (Plant) - Wheat grass is one of the best sources of living chlorophyll available, chlorophyll is the first product of light which contains more light energy than any other element. Wheat grass is very high in oxygen and beneficial to every cell in the body, rebuilds the bloodstream, and builds the red cell count. Helps hair from greying, promotes healthy skin and treats eczema and psoriasis.

Chapter 28

Cleanse and Detox Away Aging

A Time and Space for Cleansing.......
Time Cleanses Pain..... Tears Cleanses the Heart.......Solitude
Cleanses the Mind....Natural Foods Cleanses the Body......

If you take a closer look at the word "CLEANSE",
you will see the word "LEAN" hidden in plain sight. It is
no secret that people who tend to age well implement a
cleansing ritual from time to time or on a needed basis.
Leaner bodies look younger and age slower AHA!

Cleansing maximizes clean eating and supports a healthy
lifestyle. Although both cleansing and detox are similar
and are often referred to interchangeably they are
different. They are actually two different processes and
have two different purposes. The "Detox" primary
purpose is to specifically eliminate toxins (such as
chemicals, heavy metals, cigarette residue and
environmental elements) from the body by turning them
into waste to be eliminated. The objective is to enhance

the body's detoxification pathways (mainly the liver).
The liver is the body's main filtering organ.
On the other hand the "**Cleanse**" primary purpose is to
clean out the digestive tract. This process includes
eliminating toxins, fecal matter, parasites and fungi from
the digestive tract. Typical cleanses include eliminating
processed foods, sodas, refined sugars, caffeine, dairy,
gluten, soy and alcohol.

The fact of the matter is, no matter how good we plan
and execute clean eating our food sources are tainted
with pesticides and the environmental pollution we
encounter on a daily basis our bodies can benefit
tremendously from cleansing and detoxing the body of
toxins and waste that gets left behind.

How do you know if your body is toxic? How do you
know if you need to cleanse or detox? Great question!
If you suffer from headaches, joint pain, food
sensitivities, fatigue, bloating and recurring colds,
constipation, high blood pressure, mood swings, anxiety,
muscle fatigue, then without a doubt you are in need of
both a detox and a good cleanse.

There are all sorts of methods and techniques to cleanse and detox the body from fasting to consuming various foods and herbs with cleansing properties. Cleansing and detoxing does not mean you have to starve yourself in fact you should still follow clean eating habits and a good detox or cleanse is one that you can implement and support your current lifestyle.

In most cases you will have to change a few eating habits but it should not be anything extreme or drastic as your body could react adversely. Please discuss any change in your diet with your doctor first.

Below are a few simplistic ways to detox and cleanse your body:
- Drink water alone or water + lemon/lime pinch of cayenne pepper
- Oil Pull with coconut oil or sesame oil (swish around and spit out)
- Drink Cranberry Juice
- Drink Prune Juice
- Drink Detoxing Herbal Teas (Burdock root, Chicory tea, Ginger tea, Guduchi tea, DandelQion tea, Fenugreek tea, Neem tea,

Manjistha tea, Red Clover tea, Gymnema Sylvestre tea)

- Colonics
- Mag O7 (Magnesium that has been ozonated)
- Fasting (not starvation, but allowing your body a break from digesting meals) discuss with your doctor if you have diabetes or any other personal health issue before fasting.

Chapter 29

Ageless Essential Oils

Aging is Essential So Don't Be a Tin-Man.... Being Stiff is Reserved for Our Finale..... Loosen Up Add a Little Oil.....

Essential oils are wonderful for so many reasons. The most obvious of course are their natural beautiful scents. These oils are easily looked over as just being air fresheners or often equated with some kooky hocus pocus snake oil used in mysterious ways. Essential oils have been used for centuries to heal, preserve health, and beauty. There are many oils that improve our health in many natural ways.

Before opting for those extreme measures to treat those laugh lines or your furrowed brows. Try some of these natural oils that go deep into the skin to cleanse, moisturize heal and prevent many signs of aging.

- **Palmarosa oil:** hydrates and assist in skin renewal along with antiseptic properties

- **Black Seed Oil:** anti-aging, moisturizes skin, anti-inflammatory, essential fatty acids and amino acids and vitamins.
- **Neroli oil:** regenerates skin cells and increases skin's elasticity
- **Frankincense oil:** tones and lifts skin and improves fine lines and wrinkles, fades skin discolorations
- **Chamomile oil:** calms skin irritations, repairs skin and reduces puffiness around eyes
- **Cypress oil:** helps to reduces puffiness around the eyes and antiseptic properties
- **Rose oil:** moisturizes and hydrates skin acts as a barrier
- **Myrrh oil:** helps to prevent tissue degeneration
- **Rosehip Seed oil:** natural form of retinoic acid (vitamin A); exfoliates skin
- **Sea Buckthorn oil:** antioxidant rich, helpful with skin disorders such as acne, improves skin discolorations and tightens pores
- **Carrot Seed oil:** skin detox properties, nourishes tightens and rejuvenates skin

- **Geranium oil:** tightens skin, heals bruises, broken capillaries and helps to restore burned skin

- **Lavender oil:** helps to relax resulting in favorable conditions for the skin and regenerates mature skin and heals scarring

- **Tea Tree oil:** fights bacteria penetrates many layers of the skin preventing breakouts, heals acne and insect bites

- **Jojoba oil:** all in one oil, smooth wrinkles, excellent emollient, very similar to natural sebum in human skin

- **Ylang Ylang oil:** helps control oil production, regenerate skin cells and improves skin texture and elasticity

- **Helichrysum Oil:** protects skin from free radicals, anti-aging properties, wound healing and skin cancer protectant.

- **Emu Oil:** essential fatty acids (omega3s), improves skin texture, reduces fine lines and reduce the appearance of scars, burns and stretch marks.

Chapter 30

7 Habits of The Ageless Lifepreneuers

You Are What You Eat....But We Become Creatures of Our Habits.....

We all have heard of entrepreneurs of course, as many of us have anchored and set our sails toward the island that pays top dollar for ingenuity, hard work and turning a dollar into a dream. Entrepreneurship is highly respected in today's society. We look to people who have started small businesses and flourished as a result of their dedication, hard work, determination, vision and can do spirit. It is really the new American Dream as others have been inspired to follow suit. Well we all may not be cut out for business entrepreneurship, but we definitely can take that same enthusiasm in the ownership of creating and designing our own LIFE. I like to refer to it as being a "LIFEPRENEUR". My definition of a Lifepreneur is one who takes full ownership in personally investing in the business of their LIFE.

1   Develop A Deeper Connection With Their Higher Power

Almost all happy, healthy, people who appear to be ageless have formed a well-defined personal bond with their creator. You cannot love life and fear aging. You must accept what you cannot change. However, every day you can live in your acceptance and work with what you have and where you are. You only get one body this go around treat it as your temple and it will serve you well throughout your life. Connecting with your source and taking care our earth suit while we are here in the physical, protecting our mind, feeding our spirit all enhances our ageless spirit.

2   Eat Healthy and Exercise

Ageless beautiful bodies eat healthy and exercise there is no getting around living a holistic healthy lifestyle. Many have tried to cheat it, go around, under, and even jump over it only to run into health issues and obstacles that prevent them from their objectives and goals to live healthier. The ultimate goal is to be healthy not just lose weight or fit into those favorite jeans. Of course losing that extra weight is always good for our vital signs.

There is so much more to weight than the eye can see. Our thoughts manifest in our body image. If you think you are not enough or you are holding any kind of negative thoughts of yourself, it will manifest itself in your health blueprint. Emotions manifest in our body weight. Sporadic food binges are tied to our emotions and our urge for instant gratification or quell our emotional wounds of hurt and suppress the pain we all experience in our lives. When you uncover your emotional triggers you will fully be conscious of your eating habits. Not eating a diet rich with nutrient foods manifest in unhealthy weight gain and or weight loss. The healthy and ageless strive for the tree of life which is health and wellness not just a branch, bark or leaf off the tree of life. Health and wellness connects all the aforementioned into our health blueprint for success.

3   Subscribe To Preventative Health Practices

The best practice for real health is staying on top of any health issue that may arise. Of course we never know what is in store down the road. But we all know bad habits such as smoking, drinking, consuming too much sugar, over eating, salting our foods and not exercising is setting ourselves up for bad health down the road. Also we can prevent or slow some conditions by keeping abreast with our annual exams. Keep those annual appointments they serve as a baseline for your health and wellness it allows you to see where you are today compared to previous years. As well as preventive measures help in the event of any unforeseen issues with your health as time is a big proponent in various treatment options. Eating healthy food is like taking our daily dosage of medicine versus bad health forces our hand to take prescribed drugs when our body is in dire straits and under attack. Medication can be natural and medicinal or it can be drug induced. We do not want the latter as it is unnatural and the body breaks down overtime with synthetic drugs. Think of high nutrient foods as natural medicine and the drugs the doctors prescribe more times than not as drug relief. One is taken to stave off disease and the other is taken subsequent to disease.

4   Do Not Allow Age to Dictate Living a Purposed Life

Many have allowed society to dictate their reality. If society says your middle aged at 40 many will accept this sight unseen. The truth is when you live a healthy lifestyle you are as young as your daily habits you practice. Age does not have to set the bar on how you feel about yourself. It does not mean you have to lose your enthusiasm for living an inspired life. Live in your moments of joy, happiness, contentment knowing that you are aging to perfection. Aging does not have to be a daily reminder of health challenges or even death. View aging as more time to live out your purpose here on earth. Never count your days in years. Life should be counted in daily moments, breathes, I love you's, good mornings, good nights, happy borndays, happy mother's days, giving, caring and celebrating our daily blessings.

5   Invest in Health and Wellness and Make it a Top Priority

We can find the time and resources for things we think are important. We enjoy living in our beautiful home, driving our nice stylish cars and paying a pretty penny for a closet full of clothes. A lifestyle to anyone on the outside looking in would appear perfect. There is absolutely nothing wrong with living a life well deserved from all of our hard work. Enjoying the fruits of our labor is great! By all means we all should have the things we need first and desire a lifestyle nothing short of fabulous. But your health should never come in last place or compete with any of those luxuries. Health is not a luxury it is a necessity to live your ultimate lifestyle. If you don't put yourself at the top of your lifestyle to include exercising the body and accessing your wellbeing on a daily basis you are setting yourself up for some pitfalls. True wealth should always incorporate your health. If you are working your fingers to the bone, at least keep those bones healthy. Working for the sake of money alone, the by any means to an end lifestyle comes with a huge price at the expense of your health that you could never afford. You cannot fully enjoy your life if you have to suffer with poor health. Invest in your health on all levels and reap all the rewards of living your highest quality of life. For some this could mean joining a gym, creating your own space at home, taking time for yourself, building a stronger spiritual connection, parking the car walking more, eating more fruits and vegetables, investing in a nutritional system that can sustain your lifestyle or all the above. The absolute best investment you could ever make is in your health. The rewards far outweigh any physical or monetary gain. No matter how much money you earn you will never have real wealth without health. There will always be opportunities to earn more money this is not the case with our health. Health is a peace of mind not afforded to everyone.

6 Take Measures to Renew, Rejuvenate and Relax The Mind Body and Soul

Hey we all know how stressful living life can be. We can get pretty overwhelmed with life's "TO DO's" and life's "DON'T FORGETs" along with life's "I DON'T HAVE ENOUGH TIME IN THE DAY's". But where is your "TAKE CARE OF YOURSELF" 1st list? Take the time you need to relax and release and restore. It's all about leveling up daily. Set some quiet time aside for your needs to pull yourself back together after being torn in so many different directions. Make that spa or hair appointment, take that much needed walk and spend some time outside away from everything and everybody. Our rest breaks gives us that second wind we need to keep going to keep running our race. It recharges our spirit, mind and body.

7 Feed The Brain Keep Learning and Aspiring to Personal Growth and Development

If you leave a garden idle the weeds will grow this environment is not conducive for flowers and plants to flourish and grow freely. The same analogy applies when we allow our mind to become idle. Our mind is the source and power that God gives us to create and manifest our physical life. Be a lifelong learner! The learning keeps us young at heart and keeps us yearning for a new day. Allowing your mind to be overrun by weeds starts our bodies decline. All things start in the mind. Eating rich nutrient foods helps to physically feed our brain but our brain requires food for thought as well. Having an ageless body can be attributed to the mind of that person. Mind over matter is more than an expression when trying not to eat the cake, pizza or ice cream and opting for the veggies and protein shake.

We can employ mind over matter with our entire life including how we view growing older. Keep a young healthy mind and you will surely age slower than those who leave their mind open to idle distractions and allow any and everything to enter. Not guarding your mind creates a formidable obstacle in aging gracefully. You must take control of the very thing that can age you faster than time itself.

Chapter 31

Eat To Thrive

Plant Base Foods +Fruits + Vegetables + Fish + Vitamins + Oxygen Foods+ Water (H2O) = Healthy Lifestyle Blueprint......

Maintaining a healthy lean body is key to looking youthful at any age. Our bodies were made to consume the proper nutrition from natural or as close to natural food sources in order to thrive and stave off disease. The true meaning of optimal health does not end when you get that body of your dreams. Being healthy is your body's state of being without disease, mental dexterity and spiritual growth. Many people view health through the eyes of what the body looks like on the outside. The physical shape of your body does not dictate what is going on internally.

There are many types of diets. When I use the term "diet" I am not speaking of "dieting" I am speaking of diet as in the nutrients we habitually consume in order to survive. Vegan, vegetarian, fruitarian, we eat to live not for pleasure or to fill various voids in our lives. Below are various categories of special diets that are based mostly on plants, botanicals, fruit and fish with very little consumption of red meat.

- **Plant Based diet:** Mostly vegetarian and fruits are consumed and some may eat fish
- **Flexitarian diet:** Mostly vegetarian diet and occasionally meat is consumed
- **Pescetarian based diet:** A diet that includes fish but not meat

Everything we consume shows up on our body or there will be some indicators good or bad internally. The foods we eat act as fuel, the better the food source the better our bodies will thrive and perform. If we look at our body as an automobile, each car has a different type of fuel needed in order for your car to run as designed. The exact same thing goes for our body. You have 87, 89 and 93 Supreme. Your car can ride with any of these types of gas however, your car runs better on the gas specifically designed for your vehicle. We can eat a whole lot of foods and food like substances but there are natural foods that are more digestive friendly for our body's eco system. Food that is planted, sprouting from the ground or growing from trees and fish found in the ocean's water. These food sources are our body's premium fuel.

Whether you are a vegetarian or a meat eater, implementing fruits and vegetables into your diet is vital to maintain healthy cholesterol levels, blood pressure, cardiovascular health, blood sugar and glucose levels. Fruits and vegetables are filled with oxygen one of the most important elements that supports our life source. The body can survive without water and food for a few days but a second without oxygen and the body begins to shut down. Oxygen plays a vital role, not only in our breathing processes but in every metabolic process in our bodies. Our cells need oxygen to release the energy from the food we consume. By taking in more oxygen into the body our body becomes revitalized and operates at a healthier state of being.

You may be thinking you have never seen foods with a percentage label of oxygen listed. And this is due to the fact foods with a high concentration in oxygen do not come with labels such as fruits and vegetables.

Eating more of the foods listed below will improve oxygen levels in your body:

- **Lemons:** A simple twist of a lemon provides very high levels of oxygen and electrolytes into the bloodstream

- **Alfalfa Sprouts, Apricots and Sweet Apples:** These veggies and fruits are very high in fiber with a pH level of 8 and rich in oxygen

- **Legumes:** Includes peas, dry beans, and lentils helps the body process oxygen and has a significant amount of protein

- **Sardines and Salmon:** Oxygen promoting and source of lean protein

- **Water (H_2O):** Water is vital for oxygen to flow throughout the body and reach vital organs and cells

- **Vitamin A:** Makes oxygen carrying blood cells

Chapter 32

Anti-Aging Super Food Smoothies

24 KARAT GOLDEN MILK SMOOTHIE

1 ¼	Cup of Water
2 tsp	Almond Cashew Butter
1 tsp	Coconut Oil
1 tsp	Turmeric
1 tsp	Ginger
1 tsp	Cinnamon
1 tsp	Vanilla Extract
1 tsp	Honey
1	Frozen Banana

Mix Almond Cashew Butter + Coconut Oil, Turmeric, Ginger and Cinnamon Add Water and Frozen Banana Blend until smooth

Blend all ingredients with ice until smooth

- Improves digestion & bloating
- Promotes glowing skin
- Fat Buster

PINEAPPLE PARSLEY SMOOTHIE

¾	Canned Coconut Milk
¼	Fresh Chopped Parsley
1 tsp	Lime Juice
1	Can of Frozen Pineapple Chunks
½	Cup of Water

Blend all ingredients until smooth

- Improves digestion
- Promotes wound healing
- Lessens arthritis pain
- Treats colds and cough

GREEN PEACH SMOOTHIE

¾	Cashew Milk or Hemp Seed Milk
½	Plain Greek Yogurt
1 tsp	Spirulina Powder
1 tsp	Lime Juice
1	Cup of Frozen Peaches
1	Handful of Spinach

Blend all ingredients with ice until smooth

- Promotes weight loss
- Lowers hypertension
- Aids in blood sugar level
- Helps with anemia

MATCHA MINT CHIP SMOOTHIE

1 tsp	Matcha Powder
1	Cup of Almond Milk
1	Slice of Avocado
3-4	Leaves of Fresh Mint
1	tbsp. Cocoa nibs
1	Frozen Banana

Blend all ingredients with ice until smooth

- Antioxidant boost
- Weight loss
- Digestive cleanse
- Lowers cholesterol
- Protects cells

BEET RASPBERRY BLIZARD/with CHERRY ON TOP SMOOTHIE

¼	Cup of Grated Beet Root
¾	Cup of Frozen Raspberries
	A Squeeze of half Lime/Lemon
1	Cup of Unsweetened Almond/Cashew Milk
1	Scoop of Vanilla Plant Based Protein Powder

Blend all ingredients with ice until smooth

- Detoxes liver
- Keeps you satiated
- Rich in fiber
- Anti-inflammatory
- Builds muscle

Chapter 33

Whole Foods + Quality Supplementation

Natural Whole Foods + Supplements = Optimal Health & Longevity.....

Supplements are required and a must especially as we age. Batman is a pretty good superhero on his own but with Robyn as his sidekick it makes the crime fighting duo in a league all their own. Well it's the same for eating a healthy well-balanced diet. The fact still remains if we want to fight disease and achieve our maximum life span unfortunately, we can't do it on diet alone. This is where proper healthy supplementation comes to our rescue.

Supplementing a well-balanced diet will promote optimal health and wellness as our bodies endure the forces of aging, gravity and stress. So what are supplements actually and why do we need them? Supplements are derived from whole food sources or are man-made in a laboratory and manufactured and sold on the market to assist the body in a variety of ways. Vitamins are a common well known form of dietary supplement other supplements exist in the form of herbs, protein shakes, electrolytes, spices and foods. Supplements are not a substitute for natural whole food sources in your diet. I mean you would not consume 85% of supplements and 15% of natural foods. Supplements merely act to augment your diet with nutrients you are unable to absorb via consuming natural foods due to a variety of reasons. A multivitamin is recommended as a baseline to ensure you are receiving proper amounts of vitamins and minerals daily. Special supplements act to address specific vitamin deficiencies and health issues. Supplements are typically related to health and nutrition as a daily plan or supplements exist for peak performance outside normal everyday use such as professional athletes and bodybuilding. Supplements exist far and wide across many consumer needs.

Before using any supplement it is important to speak with your health care provider to assess your dietary needs. Supplements can provide a quick and easy way to get a jump on your health and wellness. If you decide to use a supplement look for natural plant based ingredients to include superpower foods, botanicals, algae, herbs, fish oils, vitamins, minerals, fruits, greens and the highest natural source of protein.

Read the labels understand the benefits different supplements provide and what common issues they can possibly treat or side effects if any are noted. Many supplements on the market have ingredients with adaptogens and plant botanicals. Adaptogens are a unique class of healing plants that help our bodies restore, balance and favorably adapt to stress at a cellular level. Botanicals are plant based ingredients that offer vitamins, minerals and amino acids that promote health and wellness.

Consuming some of the following adaptogens and botanicals will boost your body's ability to heal and normalize your stress levels. Many adaptogens can be found in your local grocery store. Supplements can also be very beneficial in combining many ingredients into one product versus buying each ingredient separately which optimize absorption into our body such as a supplement that offers a prebiotic and probiotic in one capsule.

Alfalfa: Is a plant that roots extend 20ft-30ft below ground level and brings minerals to the surface, for this reason it is known as the father of all plants. Rich in vitamins and minerals contains protein, vitamin A, vitamin B1, vitamin B6, vitamin C, vitamin E, vitamin K, calcium, potassium, carotene, iron and zinc.

Benefits: Promotes healing of the kidneys, relieves fluid retention and swelling, treats auto-immune disorders, treats arthritis, nourishes the digestive, skeletal, glandular and urinary system, cleanse the blood and bowels.

Aloe Vera: A juice or gel from the leaves of the liliaceous plant. Aloe Vera is extremely rich in nutrients and antioxidants. High concentrations of vitamin A, vitamin B, vitamin B2, vitamin B3, vitamin B4, vitamin C, vitamin E, folic acid, choline, calcium, iron, potassium, copper, manganese, selenium, sodium and chromium.

Benefits: Improves digestion, promotes internal and external healing, fosters weight loss, supports detoxification, boost immune systems and reduces inflammation.

Astragalus Root: Astragalus is a powerful adaptogen. Astragalus has an abundance of anti-aging properties as well as saponins, flavonoids and polysaccharides.

Benefits: Uses your body to produce more telomeres, contains a special class of polysaccharides which are very biologically active, improves the rate of replication of immune cells called macrophages. The gradual shortening of telomeres as aforementioned is an important component of ageing and different types of cancer. Astralagus is a powerful adaptogen that aids in preventing the shortening of telomeres.

Bieberstein's Carlin Thistle: A European perineal plant similar to Dandelion.

Benefits: Promotes detoxing of kidney and aids in stomach issues, combats fever by strengthening the immune system, heals sores and scars.

Plant Based Enzymes: Enzymes are essential to life. A superfood they treat many health maladies. Proteases: Peptidases, Trypsin, Chymotrypsin, Elastase, Bromelain and Ficin.

Benefits: Promotes healthy digestion (gas, bloating, GERD, reflux, heartburn and irregularity). Crucial to the breakdown of protein in the body

Rhaponticum (Maral Root): Contains very high amounts of antioxidants and flavonoids, natural sterols and a powerful substance known as 20-Hydroxecdysone. Maral root is loaded with tannis, glycosides, alkaloids and organic acids.

Benefits: Replenishes strength and energy, restores mental awareness, increases lean muscle mass and helps decrease fatty tissue, reinforces contractions in the heart muscles.

Rhodiola: (Golden Root or Artic Root)
Rhodiola increases the body's ability to handle stress of all kinds. It tones down the sympathetic (fight or flight) nervous system and increases the relaxing parasympathetic system.

Benefits: Prevents negative impact of emotional stress, improves endurance levels, shortens recovery time after strenuous exercise, increases attention span and improves mental keenness, decreases the amount of adrenaline and cortisol released during stress, supports fat loss, optimizes serotonin and dopamine and other neurotransmitters in the brain and prevents the development of hypoglycemia.

Schizandra (Schisandra): A powerful adaptogen that allows the body to balance physical and mental stress. Contains very high levels of antioxidants such as (Gosmin A and Wuweizisu C), protects your cells from free radical scavengers in the body.

Benefits: Increases energy at the cellular level, fights fatigue, protects and detoxes liver, aides in treating Hepatitis C.

Gogi Berry (WolfBerry): Dried goji berries contain calories, carbohydrates, fat, dietary fiber, sugar and protein. Gogi berries are very high in good sodium, potassium, calcium, iron, zinc, selenium, vitamin C, carotene, thiamin, riboflavin, lutein, lycopene, zeaxanthin, polysaccharides, betaine and peptidoglycans.

Benefits: Beneficial in lowering and controlling diabetes, promotes healthy cholesterol, prevents free radical scavenging, protects the cardiovascular system, liver functions and brain cells. Wolfberry creates a sense of well-being.

Chapter 34

Conscious Awareness of Healthy Living

The Universal No No's that impede a healthy lifestyle. .....

True health and wellness is reinforced by being cognizant of the factors that derail your health journey. The above chapters are all examples on how food, thought, exercise, sleep, self-love, gratitude, prayer and supplements can improve and change your lifestyle. Your ability to replace your existing bad habits with healthy choices creates a healthier lifestyle. Your results are directly connected to your level of receptiveness to learn and be open to healthy change. Many people love the taste of food. I am certainly one of those people. There is no reason to give up on taste. There are plenty of healthy options to enjoy without sacrificing the taste of your food. The good news is that every day will not be a protein or green shake day. You do not have to reduce your lifestyle to a liquid diet. There is no need to drink green shakes from dawn to dust. Learning new ways to be creative in the kitchen and being flexible to try new recipes will change how your mind and body receives food. Once you develop the habit of clean eating you start to acquire the taste for healthier food. Look for opportunities to improve your eating habits. For some this may mean cutting out all sodium, processed foods, sugars and soda's and fast foods. Some will decide to go meatless or live a total vegan lifestyle. For other's it may mean keeping their existing eating habits and doing more exercise and implementing a cleansing regimen. But no matter where you fall on the spectrum as far as improving your health the list below are major health destroyers that should be eliminated from your daily lifestyle.

The following are a list of toxic habits with a corresponding alternative option to support your transition to a healthier lifestyle blueprint.

Salt: Substitute with sea salt or Pink Himalayan or spiced seasoning that does not contain table salt.

White Sugar: Substitute with pure honey, cane sugar, or sweeten with natural sources of fructose such as molasses or even dark chocolate (starting at 70%), Stevia from the leaf and Monk fruit juice (which is naturally sweeter than refined sugar).

Fried Foods: Substitute with raw, grilled, or baked foods.

Fast Foods: Start a food prep, substitute with protein shakes, meal replacement shakes or energy protein bars, fruit and water.

Bad Fats: Substitute with good essential fats, eat nuts, cook with olive oil, coconut oil, avocado oils.

Sun Exposure: Keep sun exposure to a minimum, always protect your skin while outdoors with a sunscreen SPF 30+ or higher, add vitamin D3 to your diet regimen.

Stress: Look for ways to reduce stress, exercise, sing, dance, read a book, look in the mirror smile, write a letter to an old friend, Give thanks and praise God to be alive.

Negative Thoughts: Stop stressing, replace negative thoughts with positive imagery, speak powerful declarations and affirmations out loud, view your life in its totality and not just from a particular circumstance.

Obesity: Eat well balanced meals to include healthy natural lean sources of protein, fruits and vegetables. Don't forget to drink water. Also include the most natural quality supplementation where needed. Exercise daily to include cardio and resistance and strength training exercise, cut out sugars, starches and processed foods and get your proper amount of sleep.

Radiation in Food: Substitute by eating raw food and/or preparing and cooking food via conventional oven or stove top methods. Say goodbye to the microwave lifestyle. Take the time required to prepare and eat food properly. Don't think of it as wasting time in the kitchen, think in terms of adding the time that really matters and counts towards your new healthier lifestyle.

Alcohol: Substitute with red, purple, white wine, however do not over indulge.

NO SMOKING!!!!!!

NO DRUGS!!!!!!!

END OF STORY!!!!

My PRAYER for you is that God extends you Joy, Abundance and Prosperity over all your days..........

My WISH is that all of your Blessings out number all the stars in the sky..........

My HOPE for you is that you will take care of yourself to reap all of your blessings God has ordained over your LIFE!..........

GOD BLESS,
~ Coach Renatta